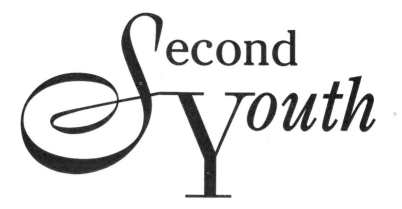

Second Youth

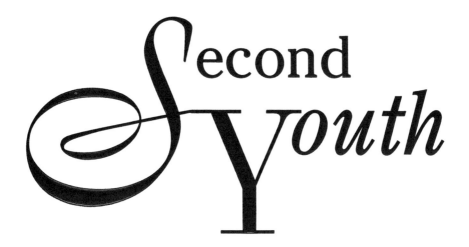

Second Youth

VERNICE GABRIEL

with
JEANNE MOLLI

Instant Improvement, Inc.
New York

The intent of this book is solely informational and is in no way meant to be taken as nutritional or medical prescription. Please consult a health professional should the need for one be indicated.

Instant Improvement, Inc.
210 East 86th Street
New York, New York 10028

Front Matter and Jacket Design — Sam Magee
Design and Typesetting — Bill Magee
Exercise Illustrations — Bob Barnes
Editor — Roberta Waddell

Printed in the United States of America

Fifth printing, 1998

Library of Congress Cataloging-in-Publication Data

Gabriel, Vernice.
    Second youth / Vernice Gabriel with Jeanne Molli.
        p.   cm.
    ISBN 0-941683-32-X
    1. Middle aged women – Health and hygiene.   2. Middle aged women – Nutrition.   3. Longevity.   I. Molli, Jeanne.   II. Title.
RA778.G23   1995
613'.04244 – dc20   95-7944

Contents

Part 1

Part 2

Part 3

About the Author

*M*any people tell me it is too late to start a new career, but I have led many lives and had many careers — why should I stop now? I have at least 40 years ahead of me. That should be enough to mold a character or two! There are no barriers that are insurmountable!"

—*Vernice Gabriel*

Picture this, dear friend–

Vernice Gabriel, an ex-fashion model, who, in her 40's, had allowed herself to age beyond her years. Desperate and aging far too fast, she staked everything on discovering — through her at-home research — a source of foods that erase those years of aging, a natural source of Young Woman's Hormones. Now, her triumph gives you thirty extra years of Second Youth.

Only twelve years ago, this same woman, formerly a top fashion model, had allowed herself to grow old and fat. Her complexion was gone. Her figure was bloated. Her body was suffering the first agonies of menopause.

Doctors were no more help to her than they are today to you. In despair, she turned to Nature. For years, she read everything written on natural healing. On menopause-defeating foods and supplements. On age-defeating foods and supplements.

She Found Over 100 of These Second Youth Foods

Once she used these *age-repair foods*, years melted away from her face and figure, month by month. Puffiness disappeared from her face. Dark circles vanished from under her eyes. The natural glow returned to her cheeks. 62 pounds of ugly fat melted away. Lines that were beginning to etch themselves across her face, halted, were stopped dead in their tracks, and slowly, week after week, began to fade from sight.

As if by magic, the vitality she had as a young woman was restored to her body. Where once she could hardly pull herself out of bed, suddenly she was bursting with energy and could once again be in front of the camera all day, and still spend half the night at dinner, the theatre, and dancing. Within months, whenever she entered the room for dinner or a party, her friends rushed over to her, gasping with amazement. "What happened to you," they said. "A face-lift? It couldn't have been just another spa! If he's a young lover, give me his phone number. If you made a pact with the devil, sign me up, too."

Within six months, she looked like her own daughter. Here was a woman who at 47, looked 60 . . . and now, at 59, she looks barely more than 35. Younger men began to pursue her. Her clothes became two or three sizes too big for her — clothes she once thought were going to imprison her for the rest of her life — and had to be given away to the Salvation Army.

Her hair took on brilliant new shine and glowed with luster. Her eyes sparkled. The skin all over her face and body firmed up, and no longer did she have to avoid the beach, or shun dresses that had no sleeves.

Now, when she walks down the street with her daughter, people relate to them as though they were sisters. At one point, she went out with a man who is three years younger than her daughter. She uses less and less makeup, because there is less and less to disguise and hide. Age moved backwards for this woman, and the results are breathtaking.

No doctor was involved in this transformation. No surgery. No Collagen. No pharmaceuticals. Only foods and supplements, exercise, and a change in mental attitude. Age-repair foods and supplements. Age-erasing exercise. Years-evaporating mental attitudes.

And — perhaps most important — her health soared. Where before she was a victim of arthritis, headaches, and almost unbearable nervous tension, now all of these have blissfully vanished. Even the colds that plagued her both summer and winter no longer can gain a foothold in her body.

At her last medical checkup, her doctor confirmed once again that she has 25-year-old bones, in a body that he would validate is more 25 years old than 59 years old.

She spent 15 years learning how to be young again. How to enjoy, not middle age, but Second Youth. How to go from flabby to firm. How to go from faded to fabulous. How to go from perpetually exhausted to perpetually excited. The key to all of these attainable miracles lies in knowledge. A nutritional miracle had happened to this woman.

And it opened up again for her the world of stardom. Once more her career skyrocketed — modeling, acting, movies, television, the theatre.

You may have seen her in major movies such as *Wall Street*; on soap operas; on the stage; or selling her homemade breads and pastries at Bloomingdale's gourmet foods department in New York City.

She has modeled for Revlon, Clairol, Elizabeth Arden, Wella, Simplicity Patterns, Cabot Knitwear, and many swimwear and clothing designers. She has appeared in *Vogue, Harper's Bazaar, Cosmopolitan, Mademoiselle, Seventeen,* and was cover girl for many hair and beauty magazines.

Vernice Gabriel is the only model who has gone from a model star to a

A Nutritional Miracle– How to go from flabby to firm. How to go from faded to fabulous. How to go from perpetually exhausted to perpetually excited.

192-pound disaster and then back again to a model star. *US* magazine and *Hour Magazine* on TV did a special story on her success.

Her discovery of the all-natural way to Second Youth is thrilling news — not only for this woman, but for all of us. Every super-food or super-herb or super-supplement that she used to give herself this Second Youth are available to you — at this very moment — in your supermarkets, your grocery stores and your neighborhood health food stores. The exercises she used are yours in the pages of this book. The mental attitudes that transformed her life can transform yours, beginning in your first ten minute session with them, in the pages of this book.

Remember, at 47 Vernice was "old", "fat" and "washed up"! At 50, she was on top of the modeling world again!

What Vernice did is not unique. Everything she did, you can do. And, you can do it better and faster and easier than she did because she's done the research for you.

Vernice says, "I promise you this. If you have faded . . . lost your looks . . . grown pale . . . fat . . . and old-looking, it is simply because you did not have the knowledge to stop the aging process. Aging is not essential. Looking old is not essential. Feeling old is not essential. The years need not leave their mark, until you are 70, 80, or 85. And maybe not until 90!"

All you need do is follow her simple directions given you in this book. Nothing else is required. Your Second Youth starts here.

Barbara & Eugene Schwartz
Instant Improvement, Inc.

Introduction

 here is no one answer to the question of what makes a person appear to be much younger, healthier and more vital than their chronological age dictates. We are a complex species which is affected by how we take care of our mind, body, emotions and spirit. When one of these components is out of kilter, the rest suffer. I have been on a quest, since the approach of my 50th year, to bring my life into balance.

Some of the facts have come through my deliberate search for a better quality of life and some (particularly the outer image) came from my need, from childhood on, to compete in society's game of acceptance.

I had 5 strikes against me, but I wouldn't give up! (1) I was a skinny, scraggly little girl with no sense of belonging to the human race. (2) Because of poor nourishment as a child, I developed rickets, which created curvature of my spine, a concave chest, and knock-knees. (3) My mother, God bless her, died from tuberculosis at 27 years of age. (4) At 50, I contracted such a severe case of arthritis that it was sheer agony to even turn my head. (5) In my mid-forties, I had swelled from a size 8 at 115 pounds to a size 18 at 192 pounds. That was 42 lbs. more than I weighed when I was 9 months pregnant with my son.

But I never lost faith that Mother Nature had the miracles I needed . . . if I could just find them.

Let me prove to you that I most certainly did!

I became aware that my survival was dependent on my appearance, my personality and my ingenuity. So I studied the popular girls to learn what made them so well-liked. I studied the characters in movies to see what made them desirable and I set out to make myself over by reading any magazine article or source I could get my hands on that would give me the secrets of becoming beautiful.

I learned about skin care, proper nourishment; how to dress to camouflage figure flaws; how to use my hair to enhance my facial features and how to apply makeup to emphasize the best features of my face and minimize the ones I didn't like.

Another key to acceptance, that I found in my research, was a sunny personality. The people I wanted to be around were the ones who seemed to be happy with life. They made me feel good about myself and gave me the hope that life could be whatever I wanted it to be. So, I studied the principles behind their behavior and scoured every bit of material I could find on mental attitudes and spirituality.

It works! Not only in the characterlines that develop in your face over the years, but also in your health, the way you carry your body, and the overall quality of your life.

Because of poor nourishment as a child, I developed the rickets which created the curvature of the spine, concave chest, and knock-knees. But my instinct for sports and exercise enabled me to reverse the effects of these deformities by building the strength of the muscles surrounding the affected areas. I also developed a well-balanced diet that gave my body chemistry the strength to fight back.

At 50 years of age, I was tested for osteoporosis and the report showed no signs of bone loss. I also had a complete two-day-long physical examination at the age of 59 years, with comprehensive blood tests, heart tests, nerve tests, and a stress test. *All tests showed my body to be in the condition of a 25 year old!*

I started professional modeling in New York City when I was 24 years old. At that time, I was 115 lbs. and looked like a teenager. I appeared in *Mademoiselle, Seventeen* and other magazines geared to the younger generation.

However, there came the time, as I said, when I grew from a size 8 at 115 lbs. to a size 18 at 192 lbs. I was in my middle 40's and I felt my life was over. 192 lbs.!! 42 lbs. more than I weighed when I was 9 months pregnant with my son!

I didn't want to believe I was *fat*! Me, a model that clients paid a lot of money to photograph clothes on because my slender figure made their clothes look good.

I made excuses for not buying new clothes because each shopping expedition ended in deep depression. But, when I started struggling with the zippers on the 14's and 16's, I realized that I could no longer hide from reality. My figure was beginning to spread like molten lava and if it wasn't checked, I was on my way to obesity and all the dangers that go along with it.

Although I loved dancing and sports, my excuse for not participating was that I was now a lady over 40 years old. The truth was that I didn't have the energy to move my growing body and I felt self-conscious about my middle-aged spread. My self-esteem had reached rock bottom.

So, I drew on my survival techniques and turned this lemon into lemonade. I became a large-size model. That alone helped me regain my self-esteem.

However, there was another great obstacle to overcome. *Food!* How I loved the taste of it all. Eating seemed to be my most enjoyable exercise and it was very satisfying. You name it, I savored it — there was no food my taste buds would turn down. I realized I was not only eating my own meal, but, would also finish any and all leftovers at the table.

A new way of life started for me in 1984. I was reaching the half-century mark — the big FIVE-0. As I assessed what I had done with my life, I realized most of it had been spent taking care of other people and I still had dreams I had put aside.

I started losing weight through proper diet and exercise. It has been over ten years now that I have maintained my weight at 129 lbs.— size 10.

I determined to find out who I really am and what I really want to accomplish in my life. I actually started to accept myself and appreciate the things that made me different from everyone else.

I am very grateful for the person I have become. My children are grown and no longer need my constant care, so I am working toward the fulfillment of my dreams that were put on the shelf.

Life over 50 has been a new start for me and I look forward to the opportunities that the next 50 years will bring.

In your youth, your mind, body and spirit are capable of great recuperative powers but, as you get older, you believe that those powers diminish. *Not true!* As long as you have a will — and a method — to improve your life, you will find the power to make it happen.

I have found all of the above factors are necessary for my survival in society. But the major key to my real happiness and success in life is my spirituality. No matter what religion you believe in, the common denominator is that there is a Higher Power that governs your life. Some people call it instinct, talent, aptitude, luck or God. Whatever you call it, I believe that it has guided me throughout my life.

I have studied and practiced many religious beliefs and have formed my own conclusion that the Higher Power lives within me and every individual. It is universal, transcends all barriers, and is there all the time, even when you do not recognize it. We are all bound together by a common thread of inexhaustible energy, and those who tap into this Power find the ways to reach the highest potential of their life.

Whenever I felt hopeless or defeated, it was "the Power" that made me pull myself up by the bootstraps and start all over again. It showed me that there is a way if you really want to make it.

My body is the Temple for my Higher Power and, in taking good care of it, I am energized and free to reach for any goals I desire. And all those I come in contact with will benefit from my positive energy. "We are what we create!"

If you are, today, in your 40's, 50's, or 60's, I promise you that you are still young. That youth may still be buried under years of eating mistakes. But it is still there, waiting for you to revive it in a Second Youth. And this book is your guide to success.

You are never too young or too old to start a program of proper care for your mind, body and spirit. The sooner you start, the better the quality of life you will experience.

Any improvement is beneficial — you have many years ahead to live fully. Why not make them worthwhile! Every day is so precious — you can't afford to accept less than the best for even one single day.

In this book, I offer you the tools I have found to make the most of what I am. They are easy to apply and will help you to realize the true beauty and uniqueness that you are.

Anything is possible if you believe in your "Power."

Good
Luck
On
Your
Journey!
–Vernice

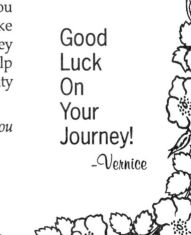

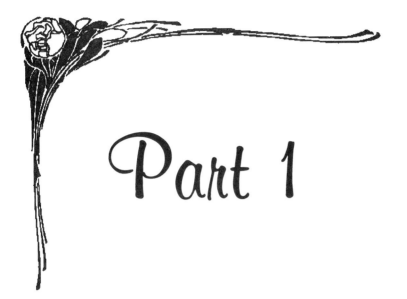

Part 1

1

How To Start
The Young Woman's
Hormones Flowing Again
In Your Face and Body

Conventional doctors call the years past 40 menopause. Far too many women call it torture. I call it meno-shift — the time in your life when you shift from your own body as the source of the *Young Woman's Hormones* to external *Super Foods* as their source.

By now, you've probably read several articles on the medical facts of menopause. All of them, of course, are accurate.

But all of them are inadequate for the kind of lives you and I wish to lead.

In brief, most doctors have no clue to the natural solution. You know too well what they say:

Your body produces the young woman's hormones until the ages of 40 or 50. Then your body shuts off those hormones, and you are left with only two medical choices. Either you take estrogen supplements, which can be disastrous, or you quickly and painfully fade into old age.

But this is too pessimistic for us. And too incomplete and unnatural for us. We say, how can your body remain old when you flood it every day with these young woman's hormones!

We say, both choices the doctors give us are, in many ways, horrendous. Either you take their pills, and become a slave to their yearly monitoring of your body against cancer. Or you accept your "natural fate," and undergo all of the tortures of hot flushes, painful sex, parchment-like skin, fragile bones, and rising heart disease and stroke risks.

So, with conventional medicine's way, you have a choice between two disasters for the rest of your life. And at this moment, you probably have chosen one or the other.

But take renewed hope! There is a third choice. *The all-natural choice*. Nature's own choice.

Now let's look at the same situation, and ask what happens to your body at ages 40 to 50 and beyond. When you ask Mother Nature, she gives you an entirely different answer: Your body no longer needs to give you these young woman's hormones. Now the plants and fruits surrounding you can furnish them for you.

Yes, when you were young, your body . . . your female body . . . was given, by nature, the precious ability to give birth. And, the first part of your life is given to you to fulfill that essential and beneficent gift. Then, when that first youth is over, nature has prepared for you the great reward for it all — your Second Youth.

Doesn't this make sense? You are now over 40 or 50. Therefore, nature knows that you have completed your child-bearing years. And, as always, she is right.

Now, at 40, or 50, or 60, or 70 or beyond, you look outside of yourself, to the bounties of nature bearing these young woman's hormones that surround you.

You can also look forward to your years of reward for the completion of that childbearing, child-rearing mission. Your Second Youth.

All the hidden safety mechanisms that nature has provided for you are there. Past cultures knew them well. Even today, sophisticated ancient cultures — which have not been corrupted by our too modern, mechanistic, artificial ways of thinking — also are perfectly familiar with them.

And all we have to do is use their knowledge to reach out and gather them in.

Let me sum it up once again. You and I have finished our first youth. We are now about to begin our Second Youth. The first came naturally from inside. The second comes — just as naturally — from outside.

In no way did nature intend for you to "dry up" when you have passed through your first youth. In no way did nature intend to deprive you of those young woman's hormones. In no way did nature say that your best years are behind you when you reach 40 or 50.

No, not at all. All nature has in mind for you is this:

When your first period of youth is over, nature simply intends for you to switch from self-production of these young woman's hormones to tapping the sources of these hormones in nature's bounteous, natural stores all around us.

I am repeating this one simple fact over and over again, because I want you to believe it as firmly as the other natural fact that the sun will rise tomorrow morning. I want it to become a part of your inner being.

I want it to be the wellspring of your central course of action from now on — reaching out to nature and getting your young woman's hormones there.

Isn't it perfectly logical? You are a part of nature. As a part of nature, there is a perfect connection between you and the rest of nature. Therefore, when you eat the right food, you turn it into new, young replacements for your own body. The food you eat, in other words, through the miracle of nature, becomes your own renewed body.

You have always known, just as your grandmothers have always known, that nature stores what your body needs in nature's many storage areas. These storage areas are known as foods.

There are foods which are packaged nourishment. There are foods which are packaged "happiness." There are foods which are "natural medicines." There are "calming" foods, "energy" foods.

And, in this chapter you will learn that there are "young woman's hormones" foods. When you eat these harmless, hormone-containing foods, you turn their power into new, young replacements for your own body. The food you eat, through the miracle of nature, becomes your own renewed body.

These are simply the foods that give you the hormones you need to have youth bloom again in your face and body. That take you back, not to your first youth, but to a longer-lasting and — even better — Second Youth.

What are these young woman's hormones? Medical scientists call them estrogen and progesterone. Just as they are found in your body, they are also found in miraculous plants and vitamins. Nature produces them, not just uniquely in the bodies of women, but also in the farms and fields.

And when your body stops producing these hormones, what is more logical and more natural than to simply go out and replace them? Yes, replace them from the herbs and plants and vitamins and minerals that also contain them.

I use Super Foods to give me the young woman's hormones that reverse the aging process. Chances are that you never heard of most of them. Used the way I show you, they take you as far beyond medicine as the jet airplane is beyond the stage coach.

And how can your body remain old when you flood it every day with these young woman's hormones?

Let me give you some examples of them.

Foods and Herbs That Contain
Young Woman's Hormones

As one noted doctor recently said, "We have proof that certain foods, rich in estrogen-like compounds, may be as effective as estrogen pills." Here are some of the best hormone restorers:

❖ *POMEGRANATES AND DATES:* These not only contain the precursors — the building blocks — of estrogens, but they contain them in packages that are also utterly delicious.

The Bible specifically mentions them for women over 40, but they've been forgotten for centuries. Take one or two of them as your mid-morning snack. This way, your snacks don't fill you with fat, but youth.

❖ *SOY FLOUR AND LINSEED:* Medical research gives startling confirmation of the young woman's hormones contained in them. For example, in England, doctors gave menopausal women foods containing soy flour and linseed as 10 percent of their daily calories for a test period of a mere two weeks.

At the end of even that short time of 14 days, when these women were tested for an "indicator of estrogen levels" circulating in their bodies, it was found to have skyrocketed 40 percent. Think of that, an increase of 40 percent in just two weeks! That's why you should have a dish of them every other day.

❖ *SOYBEANS:* Also a rich source of estrogen. Here are some soybean products:

- soybean flake
- soy grits
- soy nuts (roasted beans)
- soy powder
- tofu
- textured vegetable protein (TVP)
- soy flour
- soy milk (from cooked soybeans)
- soy oil
- soybean sprouts
- tempeh

Remember, the more young woman's hormones you eat, the more your face and body reshape themselves into those of a young woman.

Here is a startling side benefit of these soybean products

As you may have read, too much medical estrogen has now been linked to higher rates of certain kinds of female cancers.

But one noted researcher has recently discovered that eating food estrogens regularly — the exact kind we are talking about here — may actually block the runaway effects of this estrogen overload. You get all the youth benefits of their estrogens, but they actually block the cancer danger of medical estrogen.

So you obtain not only Second Youth, but protection against these terrible forms of cancer at the same moment. And this is further proven by the lower breast cancer rates in women who are vegetarians.

Understand, please, that I do not in any way suggest you become a vegetarian. I simply say that the more Second Youth foods you add to your regular diet, the more protection you get against disease.

❖ *APPLES, OLIVES, TOMATOES, CHERRIES:* More delicious fruits to enhance your Second Youth. *Caution*: figs, pineapples and pears are counter-productive, so curb your intake of them.

❖ *YAMS, POTATOES, EGGPLANT, DAIRY FOODS, MEAT:* Foods to fill the void and bring you pleasure. *Caution*: string beans, corn and tapioca are counter-productive.

❖ *ALFALFA, ANISE, GARLIC, LICORICE, PARSLEY, PEPPER, AND SAGE:* Plants, herbs, and seeds to flavor your meals. *Caution*: thyme, dill, and onions are counter-productive.

❖ *GRAINS:* Necessary in any diet for fiber and their estrogen producing properties. *Caution*: white flour, white rice, buckwheat and rye are counter-productive.

Herbs that Contain Natural Estrogen or Progesterone

- black cohosh
- false unicorn root
- lady's slipper
- life root
- passion flower

- elder
- Honduras sarsaparilla
- licorice
- Mexican wild yam
- sassafras

In addition, I especially want to mention the following:

- dong quai
- ginseng
- sage

- echinacea
- red raspberry
- sarsaparilla

How To Fit These Young Woman's Hormone Herbs Into Your Everyday Diet

Think of these herbs as rather exotic vegetables (and we will talk about some of these vegetables in just a moment).

These are forgotten herbs that contain natural estrogen or progesterone. I prefer to call the herbs "super vegetables." Therefore, they are the perfect ingredients for salads by themselves, and for side dishes at your other meals.

> Your basic rule is very simple. Mix them in with your vegetables as though they were nothing more than other vegetables.

While your unknowing or unbelieving friends around you are slipping into old age, you are aglow with Second Youth vitality, energy, attractiveness, sexuality, and slimness.

Have one or two herb and vegetable salads daily. Also cook them as a side dish for your main course for lunch or dinner.

To get an even more concentrated dosage, take one or two of them in pill form with your orange juice at breakfast. But, of course, follow the instructions on the bottle.

The point to remember with all of them is that, as Dr. George Zofchak has formally stated, "Your body will take what it needs from them, and will throw away the rest."

Where your own hormones have faded, these natural supplements take over and make the natural estrogen and progesterone flow into your body from outside your body. Their strength, their energy, their Second Youth now fuels your being.

Three Vitamins And Minerals That Really Turn On Your Body's Estrogen-Producing Power

Now you have the hormone producers. Weave at least three or four of them into your diet every day. Remember, each of them contains its portion of plant estrogens and plant progesterones. They are the Second Youth producers. Use them every day.

But there's even more good news. Recent research has shown that there is one common mineral and two vitamins that make sure you get even more of the young woman's hormones out of these herbs and vegetables. It's like adding kerosene to a charcoal fire. Everything burns brighter, and the glow you get is absolutely dazzling.

The first of these is *boron.*

This is a little-known mineral that your body needs to make these young woman's hormones. And — as an extra bonus — it also protects these young woman's hormones from being rapidly broken down by your everyday activities.

So when you take this mineral, you get more of these young woman's hormones from the foods you eat. And they keep on working for you longer and longer.

You can obtain boron in a good mineral supplement at your health food store. Take it according to the instructions on the bottle.

In addition, here are boron-rich foods that just happen to be super delicious:

- leafy vegetables
- nuts
- apples
- grapes

Have a generous serving of them every day, of course.

Now for the vitamins

Vitamin C

Take 1000 mg in supplement form every day. But, if you have not taken it before, start off with only 500 mg a day. Do this for a week and see how your body responds to the dosage. Everything should be fine, but some women have a tendency to increase bowel movements when they take larger quantities of vitamin C.

If this happens and it makes you uncomfortable, cut back to 250 mg a day. But if there is no change in your regularity, go up to 1000 mg a day. That's where you want to be — taking 1000 health-giving, youth-giving milligrams every day.

Vitamin B Complex

Vitamin B Complex is a combination of different B vitamins which are more beneficial when combined in the proper proportions because they need each other to be effective safely. Any good health food store will have several different brands. Take one a day, every day.

Also Draw Upon the Vitamin E Miracle

Vitamin E does not help you get more of these young woman's hormones out of the foods you eat. But it simply erases many of the most torturous "menopause" symptoms when it is taken in conjunction with these young woman's hormones.

For example, it helps your heart *gain* strength as you grow older, rather than lose it.

It helps your body better regulate its temperature, and therefore protects you against hot flashes.

It is remarkably effective in protecting you against lumps in your breasts, and this is essential at our ages.

It is absolutely remarkable in destroying free radicals — the runaway waste chemicals in your body that destroy your cells and tissues, and produce the worst lines and wrinkles and sags and bulges of old age.

And it is supremely powerful in fending off depression and irritability. That's why I call it my "happy pill," and always take another shining capsule of it whenever I feel that I'm descending into the dumps.

At the very least, take 100 I.U.'s everyday. I heartily recommend that within a few weeks you increase that dosage to 400 I.U.'s. That's what I take, and it makes me feel wonderful within an hour of swallowing it.

If you need a little extra shot against a particularly unhappy situation, swallow another 400 I.U.'s — that is, if you haven't had the first pill for at least eight hours. It works for me far better than a shot of liquor, and there are no — but *absolutely* no — painful side effects to fight my way through the next day.

My Bedtime Tea That Has Kept Me Away From Hot Flashes Since I Was 45

I believe that, for the past 4,000 years the Chinese knew, and still know, more about a woman's body than our highest-paid doctors today.

In China, both male and female doctors have proved that hot flashes are a minor female problem because they are so easy to deal with.

Their theory about this is very different from ours but the essential thing is that they use one of the herbs we've been talking about — *dong quai* — as a tea, or in a capsule, to treat not only hot flashes, but also the anxiety, the depression, and the insomnia that accompanies menopause for most women.

What this herb does is quite simple. It stimulates your own body's immune system to automatically self-regulate your body temperature, so those dreaded hot flashes just won't appear.

Dong quai— as a tea, or in a capsule, to treat not only hot flashes, but also the anxiety, the depression, and the insomnia that accompanies menopause for most women.

Since it's also effective at banishing insomnia — and that means it promotes natural, child-like sleep every night, without worry and without bad dreams — I drink it as a tea before bedtime.

I take one teaspoon of the powder and steep it in one-half cup of boiling water for 8 to 10 minutes. Notice that I've said only one-half a cup. That's plenty.

Also, many Chinese women add additional herbs, such as agnus-castus, red raspberry or Siberian ginseng, to the tea to gain even more and smoother benefits. Try them, too. After a short time, you'll arrive at just the right blend for your taste and body.

Incidentally, I would certainly cut down on my intake of red meat, dairy products and sugar. This is especially important if you suffer from painful hot flashes regularly.

And, this is also superb advice for anyone who wants to look and feel their best after 40 . . . in every respect.

So That's All You Have To Do!

Call it, if you will, *"The Young Woman's Hormone Feast."* Made up of daily helpings of Super-herbs and vegetables, vitamins and minerals.

A little dash here, a little sip there, and those young woman's hormones surge through your face and body again.

You are actually eating and drinking Second Youth. You are pouring it into your face and body in three delicious meals a day.

I must promise you this again: when you eat these foods, and when they furnish you with the young woman's hormones your body is crying out for now, then reversal of menopause symptoms is inevitable.

What nature has gently taken away from your body, it now supplies to your body once again, from the world of the estrogen and progesterone-producing plants all around you.

After all, if you are around 50, you still have another 35 years of health and vitality and love and grandchildren ahead of you.

First youth may have gone.
But Second Youth is better!

SUMMARY

Foods That Contain Estrogen and Progesterone

- alfalfa
- anise
- apple
- cherries
- dairy foods
- dates
- eggplant
- garlic
- grains
- licorice
- linseed
- meat
- olives
- parsley
- pepper
- pomegranates
- potatoes
- sage
- soy grits
- soy powder
- soy nuts
- soy flour
- soy oil
- soy milk
- soybean flakes
- soybean sprouts
- soybeans
- tempeh
- textured vegetable protein (TVP)
- tofu
- tomatoes
- yams

Herbs That Contain Estrogen and Progesterone

- black cohosh
- dong quai
- echinacea
- elder
- false unicorn root
- ginseng
- Honduras sarsaparilla
- lady's slipper
- licorice
- life root
- Mexican wild yam
- passion flower
- red raspberry
- sage
- sarsaparilla
- sassafras

Vitamins and Minerals That Aid Absorption of Estrogen and Progesterone

- vitamin B complex
- vitamin C
- vitamin E

Boron Found In:
- grapes
- leafy vegetables
- nuts

Caution! Avoid!

- buckwheat
- corn
- dill
- figs
- onions
- pears
- pineapples

- rye
- string beans
- tapioca
- thyme
- white flour
- white rice

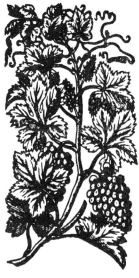

Grapes

2

From Middle Age To Second Youth

*M*iddle Age! The time in each person's life between youth and old age, usually reckoned as the years between 40 and 60.

At 59 years, I still do not feel middle-aged. My vitality, passion for living, energy and strength are just as powerful now as they were when I was sixteen. I can honestly say that this period of my life has been the most exciting for me.

Now that my children are grown and I have conquered the "empty-nest syndrome," I am finding out who I am and am working towards the fulfillment of my childhood dreams.

Now is the time to take those dancing lessons . . . craft classes . . . be a social butterfly . . . explore the world . . . read . . . write a book . . . check out the gurus in the mountains of India . . . start a new hobby . . . start a career . . . and find out what your inner self desires. The options are infinite. Follow your dreams that have been put on hold.

I chose to start an acting career at age 50. I am having a wonderful time exploring who I am and allowing the emotions that would not be acceptable in public contacts to be expressed to their fullest. Now I can cry, lose my temper, vent my anger, express my sexuality and receive the applause of everyone around me. I also take actors' movement classes that incorporate dance exercises and dances of all eras. How wonderful to feel the rhythm of my body flow with suppleness and energy to the beat of a tango, polka or waltz. And the social contact with people who have the same interests as I (no matter what their age) makes me realize I am a part of this big wonderful world.

Explore, explore — you have only one life to live and if you get out there and enjoy, you can extend it beyond what it might have been. After all, if you are about 50 yrs. old, you still have another twenty-five or thirty-five years to go if you use them actively. Remember the old adage, if you don't use it — you lose it — so what will you choose?

My children are constantly telling me they find it hard to keep up with me. My doctors marvel at the condition of my body, inside and out. They say it is equivalent to that of a 25 year old. I might even consider having another baby someday.

Middle age is a worrisome time for most people. It is the period of life when you start to feel the pressure of time creeping up on you. This is the time when you start taking inventory of your life to see if you have accomplished what you had intended and, if not, panic sets in. Youth is no longer your ally so you feel Father Time ticking away and you overstress yourself trying to beat the clock.

Unless you have maintained the best of health, your body starts to react. It begins to break down and the additional stress can result in heart attacks, ulcers, nervous breakdowns, digestive and elimination problems, poor circulation, arthritis, and on and on.

For a woman, middle age is accompanied by menopause which terminates your childbearing possibilities. Osteoporosis, a weakening of the bones caused by the enlargement of spaces or canals in the bone, makes fractures and broken bones a real risk. It generally occurs in women after menopause.

Your mind starts to ask questions that never occurred to you before the big Four-0. You start to worry about your sexual performance — will it last — will it be as exciting — will you be as attractive to the opposite sex as you used to be or will they want a younger model?

Osteoporosis, a weakening of the bones, makes fractures and broken bones a real risk.

If you are married, this is the time that you start to feel insecure in your appeal to your mate. You have been so involved with the family life that you forgot to maintain your youthful appearance. Will your mate start to seek attention from an outsider who is more youthful and exciting? It may happen, not only because you haven't held on to your youthful vitality, but also to bolster his own ego, which is just as shaky as yours.

The Joys of Sex

It is said that your sexual drive is lowered after menopause, but I have yet to see it that way. I feel the new freedom from responsibility and monthly interruptions gives rise to more desire.

Vaginal dryness can be a deterrent, but when the passion is aroused, the juices usually flow. If they fall a little short of comfort level, (don't be shy or embarrassed) use a little help. K-Y jelly, Lubifax, vitamin E oil, or any other water-soluble

> Research has proved that regular intercourse can indirectly stimulate the ovaries, moderating the estrogen level.

lubricant will ease the way. You might want to apply a lubricant before your encounter so there will be no interruption during the heat of passion. Sex is good for you, both mentally and physically.

Research has proved that regular intercourse can indirectly stimulate the ovaries, moderating the estrogen level, which reduces the hot flashes and mood swings.

Strengthening your vaginal, urinary and anal muscles can give you more pleasure during intercourse and help to prevent urinary incontinence which occurs with many of us as we get into our golden years. It is a very simple exercise that should be a part of your daily living (age is no limit), and can be done at any time, wherever you are.

Squeeze the muscles in each area as though you were trying to stop urinating or moving the bowels. Hold firmly for 10 counts and release. Repeat several times, building your holding time up slowly.

Another exercise is to hold and let go in a pulsating rhythm. Have fun doing this, perhaps even be risky and do it in public. No one will realize you are doing it, they will just wonder why you have a pleasant look or smile on your face. Be careful, this exercise can make you very horny.

When your body is functioning in *all* areas, you feel good about yourself and won't have a tendency to put yourself "on the shelf." So enjoy, enjoy! Physical contact has been known to create miracles.

Hot Flashes and Night Sweats

The lowered estrogen supply in your body is the reason for the mixed signals in your temperature-control center. Until you regulate your estrogen intake with the information given in the chapter on Young Woman's Hormones, here are some tips to make it easier:

❖ When you feel a hot flash coming on, don't panic. Remain calm and wait it out. Remind yourself that it only lasts for two to three minutes (it will seem much longer) and does not do any harm. Get yourself a lovely lace fan that you can carry in your purse and whip it out when your temperature rises. A beautiful black lace fan can be very mysterious and romantic.

❖ Drink lots of water to help your body's thermostat adjust.

❖ Vitamin C (the all-purpose vitamin) helps to regulate body temperature. Take at least 1500 mg. twice a day.

❖ Bioflavonoids boost the values of vitamin C and can be found in pill form or in the fibrous white membranes inside oranges and grapefruits.

❖ Vitamin B-complex, with B^{12} will help you ease tension and depression. They will also build your energy level.

❖ Vitamin E (d-Alpha Tocopheryl Succinate) 800 I.U. can be taken in capsule form as a supplement or you can find it in soybean oil, corn oil, wheat germ, peanuts, margarine, mayonnaise, and salmon.

❖ Selenium (200 mcg. daily) can be taken as a supplement. It is also found in asparagus, garlic, mushrooms, beef and fish.

❖ Ginseng is considered an aid to calming hot flashes.

❖ Bellergal and Clonidine are prescription medications that have been known to reduce the severity of hot flashes and night sweats. These require a doctor's watchful eye because there are side effects and contraindications that must be considered.

❖ Herbal helpers: dong quai (also called the female ginseng), Siberian ginseng, bee pollen, and primrose oil. Try a cup of tea made with sarsaparilla, red raspberry leaf, elder, black cohosh, and licorice root.

❖ Spicy foods, hot drinks, alcohol, and overeating are triggers for hot flashes so if you don't want to avoid them altogether, just sample them or treat yourself occasionally, and be prepared for the consequences.

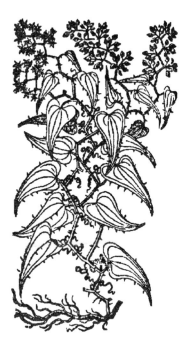

Sarsaparilla

3

What Is the Elixir of Youth?
Why Is It Desirable?

*A*H! The search for the Fountain of Youth!

For centuries, mankind has revered the properties of youth because they signify life on the verge of full bloom. The energy . . . hope . . . the promise of every possibility . . . the vitality of life . . . exuberant spirits . . . the power to survive . . . the capacity to grow, develop and accomplish . . . the powers of recuperation . . . the unbridled passions for living and loving.

Who doesn't want all of these?

Everyone wants to be happy and full of the joys of life. No one enjoys dealing with the trials of living, particularly when you feel hopeless and helpless. You have experienced all of these properties at times throughout your life but, somehow, you've lost the Essence of Youth.

Remember the high hopes you had for your life when you were young? How there always seemed to be time to work things out? There were no deadlines (excuse the pun) and if one goal didn't pan out, there was still time to start in another direction.

If a love didn't last forever — there was time to recuperate and find another mate.　45

When I was
a little girl,
I was told:

"Anything
worth having
takes an
extra effort
to make
it happen."

"A
successful,
joyful life
is not
for the
faint-hearted."

"You have
to be
a warrior
for your
ideals."

"You want
to live?
Go for it!"

You want
to feel
young
again?
You
have
the power
to do
anything!

While there
is life
there is hope!

Where there
is a will,
there is
a way!

There was the freshness of a young mind filled with eternal hope, looking out on the world as an adventure at every turn of the road.

There was the spirit that was open to trying the unknown and a body that was strong and healthy to carry you through.

This is the Elixir of Youth, the panacea that can maintain a good life indefinitely.

There is no need to explain why it is desirable. The facts speak for themselves. To have eternal youth implies that you will live forever, that your life will be full of excitement, romance and opportunities.

Well, who says you have to give them up?! You say age is creeping up on you and you have no control over the course of your life? Life has passed you by? Your body is falling apart? The mirror is no longer your friend? Romance has gone out the window? You say you're too old to start over? Your path is irreversible?

Hogwash!! All those clichés were invented by people who gave up on life. By disillusioned individuals who may have tried to live, but took the easy way out when the road got bumpy. In actuality, they created their own unhappiness by sitting back and letting come what may.

Anything is possible when you put all the "secrets" of youth into action. Start this very minute to empower yourself for the exciting road ahead. You can find your way back with the tools I have laid out for you. You can bring harmony and youth back into your life, no matter where you are on your path.

4

Secrets Of Staying Young, Healthy & Happy

*Y*es, you can call them "secrets" because when you "grow up" you forget what it was that made your youth so desirable. And when you were young, you didn't know that what you were experiencing would be so desirable when you got older.

Therefore, you go through life never documenting or acknowledging what it is that makes your life so vital and exciting. The ingredients of a youthful existence remain secrets until you are made aware of them.

Here are what I believe to be the main components of the elixir of life:

❖ MENTAL ATTITUDE: A joy in living . . . positive thinking . . . an open mind for change . . . willpower.

❖ PHYSICAL FITNESS: An active body that functions at peak performance. A well-oiled machine that responds to your demands.

❖ PROPER NUTRITION: A healthy way of eating that fuels your body. Knowing the natural ways to heal your body without chemicals.

❖ THE ABILITY TO CREATE AN IMAGE: An awareness of your outer image . . . and the knowledge to create the illusion of what you desire to be.

❖ A THIRST FOR KNOWLEDGE: Knowledge opens the world up to you and gives spice to your life.

❖ A SENSE OF HUMOR: Colors the way you see yourself and others. It gives you a different perspective on the circumstances of life.

❖ THE ABILITY TO TURN LEMONS INTO LEMONADE: Using your ingenuity to make life work for you when the chips are down.

❖ BEING IN THE MOMENT: An appreciation of life in this very moment. Seeing the beauty of even the smallest object. Feeling the emotions and rhythm of life as it is *NOW*.

❖ TAKING RISKS: Accepting the challenges that cross your path and following up on your dreams.

❖ THE ABILITY TO LOVE AND BE LOVED: The greatest gift of humanity. Without it, life is hopeless.

❖ SPIRITUAL AWARENESS: Finding the God within you and realizing your innate powers that bind you with humanity and the universe.

❖ HAVING FUN! LETTING THE CHILD IN YOU LIVE: No matter what age you are, the child you once were is still alive within your mind and body. Don't suppress her. Enjoy her!

You may realize that you have experienced each of these ingredients many times throughout your life, either singularly, in groups, or all at the same time. Those were the times you felt that life was good and you were happy.

But for most of you, those times were fleeting. You were not aware of why you were feeling so good, so you probably didn't know you could make it happen again.

Life is not easy! You have to take matters into your own hands. Be responsible for making your life work for you. Some people have forgotten how, or they were never aware of how their participation in each circumstance was detrimental to its outcome.

I have heard many people endlessly lament how poorly life is treating them. Little do they realize that they *do* have a say in the matter and must take action to make life work for them. Surely, you have seen many cases of tragedy or unbearable circumstances that have been turned around so that survival was accompanied by tremendous growth for the individuals.

Miracles? I believe you make your own miracles through believing in your own power to create a positive flow in your life. Make adversity your tool for developing your innate abilities.

In this book, I have outlined in detail the ways I have learned to make my life meaningful and enjoyable. Staying young means prolonging a good life, no matter what your age. While you are here on this earth, why not make it worth your while!

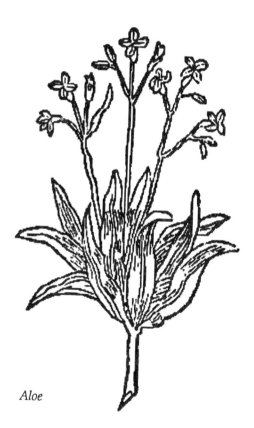

Aloe

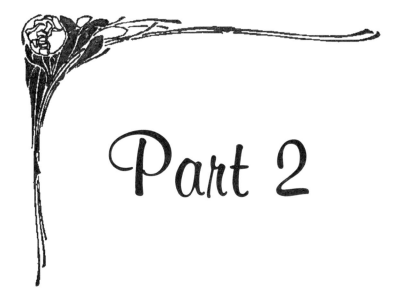

Part 2

5

Welcome to The World of Disease-Free Second Youth!

There is no faster way to age than to suffer a disease. And there is no faster way to return to Second Youth than to rid yourself of that disease . . . or prevent it in the first place.

This section will discuss the super-agers — the many diseases that plague women of our age. We will look at each one of them in turn. And we will see what natural healers can do to help you drain them out of your body.

But first, a word of explanation . . . fate was kind to me. When I had grown "too fat" and "too old" to continue modeling, I took a job in a health-book publishing firm. This was a deliberate choice on my part. When I first applied for the job, and heard what they sold — books on natural healing — I immediately jumped at the opportunity. Here was my chance to learn everything I wanted to know about the revolutionary new discoveries in foods, vitamins, herbs and sup-

Foods and nutrients out-performed the prescription drugs to which I had almost become addicted. Diseases that had plagued me for years began to slowly fade out of my life.

plements that did not require a doctor's prescription. And learn how I, myself, could make and keep myself well, without a trip to either the doctor's office, the clinic, or the hospital.

For the past 15 years that I have worked for this firm, I have been in heaven! Think of it. This firm worked with the great *Prevention Magazine* and the great new breed of nutrition heroes — Dr. William Lee, Dr. Stephen Chang, Dr. H. L. Newbold, Dr. Edward Wagner, Dr. Michael Weiner, Dr. Edwin Flatto, and many more.

I studied all their works. It was like eating candy to me — but a strange kind of "candy," that made me leaner and healthier instead of fatter and sicker.

I tried many of their latest breakthroughs. I proved, to my astonishment, that foods and nutrients could — by far — outperform the prescription drugs I had almost become addicted to. Diseases that had plagued me for years — such as osteoarthritis in my neck and chronic migraine headaches — faded out of my life.

Before I knew it, my friends were thinking of me as the neighborhood healer. I would receive phone calls from them at even 10 or 11 o'clock at night. They begged me to soothe their cramps, or take away their headaches. I became known in my circle as the "natural healer." I must have recommended, in the last five years alone, hundreds of bottles of proven vitamins, diet control, and relaxation techniques.

I have seen natural healing work for myself and for dozens of my friends. I have absolute, living proof that there are far more miracles in the right foods than there are in a dozen pharmaceutical companies.

And I especially know that this kind of proven natural healing is a godsend to the millions of women and men over 40. The women who face the growing agony and aging of what used to be called the "menopausal" years.

Chances are, if you are reading this book right now, you have (or will have) one or more of the afflictions I discuss in the following chapters. And, chances are, you have seen doctor after doctor to get help for them, and at this moment you are more than dissatisfied. Therefore, you are looking for something new, something proven, something natural, to open up new doors to health that you thought were closed forever.

Of course, I do not recommend that you desert your doctor. Far from it. All these home remedies work hand in hand with him or her. In many cases, they can even go beyond. But, at the very least, if he or she is open-minded

Natural healing miracles happen every day. They promise a disease-free, pain-free, bulge-free life for you in the next 20, 30 or 40 years. See for yourself how quick-acting and long-lasting, and above all how powerful they are.

they can greatly accelerate and facilitate the power of conventional pharmaceutical treatments.

The documentation in all the great natural healing books I have studied in the last few years shows these home remedies have worked for thousands of women. I believe they promise a disease-free, pain-free, bulge-free life for you in the next 20 or 30 or 40 years. Remember, always, that your body wants to be well. All it needs is for you to join with nature to enable it to cure itself.

Help your body heal itself. Even a doctor — any good doctor —will tell you this is the fundamental mechanism of healing. In the meantime, do not poison it. Give it the strength it needs to gather its own forces and expel the invader.

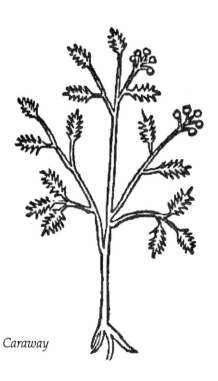

Caraway

Miracles — naturally healing miracles — happen every single day. On the following pages you will meet the finest of these that I have discovered. Try them. See for yourself how delicious, how harmless, how quick-acting and long-lasting, and, above all, how powerful they are.

6

Arthritis: How To Beat Arthritis And Have A Young Woman's Joints

Strong as your bones may be, you can still be subjected to the torture of arthritis, as I was before I found the natural healers that this chapter gives you.

Some 20 to 35 million Americans suffer from arthritis in one form or another. Rheumatoid arthritis, osteoarthritis, systemic lupus, bursitis, gout and scurvy are the known forms of arthritis. There are doctors who claim that one out of seven people feel its unremitting pangs.

Rheumatoid arthritis is an inflammatory disease in which the immune system defenders of your body attack your own tissues as if they were a foreign invader. Your joints turn to fire. They swell. They become rigid. The tissue around the joints, the skin surrounding them, and the muscles can often be affected as well . . . *and they can be treated!*

Osteoarthritis, which was my problem, is a degenerative joint disease, involving a wearing away of the cartilage from lack of lubrication. This is the most common form which gets around to almost everyone sooner or later.

❖ PERSONAL NOTE: I had to discover relief from the pain of osteoarthritis in my neck because the discs between the vertebrae had degenerated to the point where the nerves in that area were pinched and caused me a lot of pain when I tilted my head backward or sideways.

The vertebrae in my neck developed calcium deposits (spurs) that scraped the nerve trunk which comes out of the 5th and 6th vertebrae and caused an inflammation of the nerve trunk, making it swell.

Shocks of extreme pain would shoot across my right shoulder and down my arm to my fingertips. My right hand and arm would go numb for periods of time.

I was advised by doctors to have an operation, but, being a person who will try anything to avoid an operation, my alternative was to follow a therapy plan. Neck stretches to relax the cramping of the muscles and ligaments. Range of motion exercises to lengthen the shortened muscles and ligaments. Isometric exercises to strengthen the muscles that support the neck vertebrae and head. Periodic massages and *soft* chiropractic adjustments, which are most helpful. Proper posture while standing or sitting and a neck roll while sleeping are mandatory. I also wear a soft cervical collar when I sleep to prevent misalignment of my neck vertebrae when my muscles are in a deeply relaxed state.

Slight changes in my eating habits and a diet that was more nutritionally beneficial completed my course of action.

Before I found these natural healers, I was almost crippled by arthritis. Now it has been six years since my last major attack. No longer do I wake up with a headache and agonizing pain in my shoulder or arm, there are no more episodes of numbness and now I have much more freedom of movement without the slightest pain.

Now let's look at the view of orthodox medicine. The great majority of doctors still say there is nothing they can do to prevent arthritis. And there is no specific cure.

Isn't that pathetic? *The Merck Medical Manual* lists as causes: psychological stress, body chemistry problems, infectious organisms, concussion, allergic reactions, or tumors. Any one of these, according the *Medical Manual,* can be a possible instigator of arthritis.

Since there are so many possible causes, the summation of all this listing is very simple. Doctors just don't have a clue as to what really causes the disease. They admit they don't know. They don't even know where to begin to look. They are completely in the dark.

Since they don't know, their only reaction to the disease is to flood your body with a never-ending stream of dangerous drugs. These include painkillers, steroids, cortisone, etc. — all of which commonly do nothing to heal the arthritis, but do cause damaging and torturous side-effects.

Take your arthritis pain, for instance. If a doctor wants to give you "a gentle" treatment, he or she may "only" prescribe up to 14 aspirin or Bufferin or ibuprofen a day. This may diminish your pain to the point where it is barely tolerable. But it also, as you know, eats away your stomach.

So, as time goes along, you have, not one devastating disease, but two. Not only do you suffer from the torture of arthritis, but you also have developed a host of digestive ills until you end up being able to eat only baby food.

Worst of all, doctors say that treatment of arthritis by anything but these deadly drugs is "quackery." In other words, they don't know what to do to really help you, but anyone else who has an idea is automatically a fraud. There are quacks in this field, yes. But you can turn instead to the amazing nutritional discoveries made over the past two decades which freed me from the vast bulk of my arthritic symptoms and pain, and can free you as well.

Perhaps the Best Food of All for
Inflammatory Pain — a Fish!

Let's start with medical facts, with those doctors who are also visionaries of the future of natural healing. At the Brusch Medical Center in Cambridge, Massachusetts, Drs. Charles M. Brusch and Edward T. Johnson treated 100 sufferers of rheumatoid and osteoarthritis, not with drugs, but with foods. And 92 out of the 100 had less pain, reduced swelling, and far greater range of motion with the following regime:

1. They drank room-temperature milk. They had soup with their meals. They limited their water intake to one hour before breakfast.

2. They took cod liver oil at bedtime or before breakfast. They took it 30 or 40 minutes after their last drink of water for the day.

3. They limited their caloric intake to between 1800 to 2400 calories per day. If they were shorter and had a more delicate body frame, they ate 1800 calories a day. If they were taller and had a more pronounced body frame, their daily intake went up to 2400 calories. But no more. And they ate no cake, cookies, candies, sweet rolls, or other products containing white sugar or flour. And no ice cream or soft drinks.

Remember, 92 out of the full 100 had less pain, reduced swelling, and more range of motion. Isn't that worth a minor change in diet?

Now, how do you use this information? I would suggest that you immediately go on a fish diet, or take fish oil supplements.

I really recommend a hardy fish diet for anyone who suffers from any kind of arthritis or pre-arthritis-like pain. The most beneficial Omega-3 oils come from fatty cold-water fish such as cod, herring, mackerel or salmon. If you want variety, substitute swordfish and more exotic fish. The English really knew what they were doing when they served kippers for breakfast! But if you don't have time to prepare a meal like that in the morning, catch up with your fish at lunch or dinner three times a week. Try this for three weeks as a test and I guarantee you'll feel so much better.

If you have an aversion to eating fish, if you just don't like its taste, then take fish-oil supplements. They're called EPA's and you should start with a 500 mg dosage. Take one every day. If you have any doubts about going on them, and I have none, then by all means do check with your doctor. Make sure he or she is a progressive, modern visionary and he or she will have no objection at all.

Arthritis-Fighting Herbs and Spices

Ginger is often recommended for the pain and inflammation of rheumatoid arthritis. I want to stress that this is specifically for the pain and inflammation of rheumatoid arthritis. Dr. Krishna C. Srivastava of the Institute of Odense in Denmark reports that taking less than a tablespoonful every day for three months gave his patients considerable freedom from the pain and inflammation of rheumatoid arthritis.

As you know, ginger can be found in powdered form in any supermarket because we use it so often to bake with. Also, at Oriental grocers or health food stores, hands of ginger root are readily available to be peeled, chopped and

Eat fish religiously three times a week. I guarantee you'll feel so much better.

added to stir-fried dishes, or you might try my favorite, Japanese-style slivered ginger.

Then there is the Asian extract known as *rohitukine*. It can be purchased at health food stores. *Rohitukine* is an Oriental healer. One of the latest experiments with it was conducted on 30 patients for 12 weeks by Dr. A.N. Dohadwalla of Bombay. He found out that it slashes the worst effects of his patients' own immune systems turning against themselves. In other words, it greatly helps rheumatoid arthritis.

If you have pain in your knees, this paragraph is for you.

There is also a Chinese herb used for centuries, and known as Fo Ti and Ho-Shou-Wu, that is a specific for pain in your knees. And for just as long, the East Indians have valued guggul and boswellia. In fact, boswellia is used not only for the knees but also for morning stiffness anywhere in your body.

Anti-Arthritis Minerals and Vitamins

Zinc

Many rheumatoid arthritics have been found to have lower than normal levels of this mineral.

One study, at the University of Washington in Seattle, which was reported in the British medical journal, *Lancet,* showed promising results when zinc supplements were administered.

And another study, done at the University of Copenhagen in Denmark and published in the *British Journal of Dermatology* indicated significant improvement in the condition of psoriatic arthritics when given supplements of zinc oxide.

Well-absorbed food sources of zinc include herring, liver, egg yolks, soy products and peanut butter, followed by whole grains, safflower and sesame seeds. Eat them as much as possible.

Or, you should really take a good multi-mineral supplement every day. Not only for arthritic conditions, but for your general health. Most of these contain a decent amount of zinc. And if you feel better within one or two weeks after taking it, you can go up to a separate zinc supplement which contains about 15 or 20 mg of the mineral.

Anything more should be discussed with your doctor.

Copper

Again, arthritics often have higher than normal levels of copper in their synovial fluid. Rather than being seen as a bad sign, this is now interpreted as protective — especially for osteoarthritis.

This indicates, very strongly, that there is truth after all in the folk custom of wearing a copper bracelet. Why? Because copper may act as a scavenger of toxic oxygen radicals, which would therefore help your body fight off inflammatory diseases.

I certainly have nothing against bracelets of any kind — whether they be copper, gold, or diamond. However, it seems a little unlikely to me that the trace mineral copper can be absorbed through the skin from a bracelet. But if it works for you, keep wearing it.

There are, of course, dietary sources of copper. They include chocolate (what a wonderful excuse to indulge!), nuts, seafood, organ meats, dried peas, beans (also high in sulfur-bearing amino acids that strengthen the connective tissues in your joints), avocados, prunes and raisins.

The B-complex vitamins

Get these from your daily vitamin supplement, as well as from animal products, legumes and whole-grain cereals.

And then there are the old reliables, Vitamin E and Vitamin C

Vitamin E and Vitamin C

These keep the synovial fluid thin and allow greater range of movement. I take supplements of them on general principles, but they are as yet unproven as specifics for arthritis. Nevertheless, and I am going to say this again and again, you should take that vitamin supplement and mineral supplement every single day of your life (I will give you a description of its contents in a special section of this book).

Selenium

Now a specific for draining out arthritic swelling, the source of never-ending arthritic pain. Take a 100 mg a day . . . for many, many reasons.

Evening primrose oil

Evening primrose oil contributes to the manufacture of prostaglandins that have a direct anti-inflammatory action.

You can get a bottle of this at your health food store. Take one or two drops daily as instructed.

Pyridoxine

If you have carpal tunnel syndrome, the vitamin recommendation is pyridoxine (B^6). You will take it in your daily supplement. But if it shows you relief, also take a separate 100 mg a day supplement.

Folk Remedies For Arthritis — Long Maligned By Doctors — But Now Proven By Them

❖ **Yucca**. This is a member of the lily family, with broad, sword-shaped leaves and white flowers. For centuries, it was relied on by the American Indians of the Southwest as a remedy for many ailments, including arthritis. Now, Dr. Robert Bingham, who operates an arthritis clinic in Desert Hot Springs California, has proven that it certainly does relieve arthritis symptoms. Again, you can get it at your health food store. Use as directed on the label.

❖ **Hot Peppers**. For example, cayenne, chili peppers, jalapenos, paprika, etc. These also have been reputed for centuries to give relief for arthritic pain, inflammation and stiffness. They are, of course, used externally. You rub them into the skin to treat the joint pain beneath it. They contain, as their active ingredient, capsaicin, which is also sold as an over-the-counter ointment.

Why do they work? We know the answer now. They are what is known medically as counter-irritants. In other words, they distract from the deeper joint pain by providing a minor, superficial one on your skin.

This was proven again recently by a test conducted in Illinois and published in *Clinical Therapeutics*, which showed that one-third of the osteo- and half of the rheumatoid arthritis patients had considerably — that's considerably — less pain when they rubbed capsaicin cream on their knees four times daily. The rest of the 101 arthritics were given a placebo cream, and had absolutely no relief.

> One-third of the osteo- and half of the rheumatoid arthritis patients had considerably less pain when they rubbed capsaicin cream on their knees.

To make your own ointment, simply mix 1/4 to 1/2 teaspoon of dried red pepper in a cup of vegetable oil. Just apply as needed.

The Simplest Arthritis Remedy of All:
Stop Poisoning Yourself

Natural-healing doctors are now saying that, in many ways, arthritis resembles an allergy.

Let's see why. Suppose that you were allergic to roses. Every time you were in a room with them, your eyes would tear, your nose would run, all the passages of your throat would swell up until it became hard for you to breathe.

Under those circumstances, would you bring home a fresh new bouquet of roses every day, and suffer the same tortures all over again while they were surrounding you?

Natural-healing practitioners say this is exactly what you are doing with certain foods and arthritis. Because of the way your body is built, certain foods are poison to you. Other people — perhaps even members of your very own family — can eat them with impunity. For you, though, they inflict nothing but suffering.

You see, most medical, conventional doctors do not make the connection between these foods and the onset and continuance of your arthritis. They don't realize that, if you have a tomato salad for lunch, two or three hours later you can hardly move the joints of your hand because you ate tomatoes.

They don't think that food causes disease at all. To them, the cause of disease is simply and solely germs. But, in the case of arthritis, they simply can't find the germ that causes the disease.

So they are mystified. And they add poison — in the form of their drugs — to the poisons — in the form of these deadly foods — that you are already consuming.

All this is not statistically proven, of course. No drug company is going to spend millions of dollars on research to tell you to simply give up certain foods and see your arthritis pain and suffering recede. Why would they? They can't patent "giving up foods." They can't make billions of dollars a year on selling a drug that makes you give up these foods.

There's no profit for them in foods. So, instead of trying to find the truth, they try to disguise it.

But you can prove it yourself, just as I have proven it on myself, by simple dietary experimentation.

Natural-healing practitioners say that the following foods cause and inflame arthritis:

- tomatoes
- eggplant
- red and green peppers
- Irish (or white) potatoes
- tobacco

They are called Nightshades. Plants of the genus Solanum. Many of them have a poisonous juice, such as atropine, belladonna or scopolamine.

Tobacco is also a member of the nightshade family. We have all been actively warned of its effects on the body.

If taken in large quantities, these ingredients can kill you.

❖ *PERSONAL NOTE*: I honestly believe that my mother's death from tuberculosis at age 27 can be attributed to the fact that she was a chain smoker.

When I started to smoke in my late 20's, I remember the unpleasant physical sensations and reactions I experienced because my body was trying to tell me that I was harming myself. I would become dizzy and my heartrate would accelerate to the point that it was hard to catch my breath at times.

As I continued, my body adjusted to this foreign toxic invasion and eventually became addicted. I soon felt a craving for the constant supply of the nicotine.

It wasn't long before the tar residue filled my lungs and I started to cough up black phlegm. That was an obvious sign to me that my body was being damaged by my habit. I thought, if tobacco can manifest itself in this obvious way, imagine what other effects it has on my body that are not visible, and, thinking this, I immediately took steps to wean myself from the destructive pattern I had adopted.

When you eliminate arthritis allergy foods you perform a miracle on yourself. You do what no conventional doctor in the world can do for you. You stop your arthritis in its tracks.

Now, no one is going to overdose on vegetables, but eating these particular ones has been considered an aggravating factor in arthritis sufferers.

If you have either osteo- or rheumatoid arthritis, they say you are allergic to these plants, that every time you eat these plants, you feed your arthritis. You strengthen your arthritis. You inflame your arthritis. You perpetuate your arthritis.

Is this true? More importantly, is this true for you?

Why not find out? Take the two week allergy-detection test. All you do is cut out these foods for two weeks. In other words, for two weeks you have no eggplant, or red and green peppers, potatoes, tomatoes, and you stop smoking.

Do not have one bite of any of them! They are out of your life, completely, for two weeks.

Nor do you eat any products that contain them. For example, tomato sauce on spaghetti, stews and soups made with tomatoes, etc.

Just two weeks. That's all. No longer. And you will know.

You will know whether you are allergic to those foods. Because, in those two weeks, your body will have had time to get rid of all their traces. It will free itself of their residues. Or, perhaps for the first time in your life, you will be freed from any of the chemicals they contain.

See how you feel then. Has the swelling gone down? Has the pain subsided? Are you less stiff in the morning? Do you have more general energy? Do you sleep better at night, and can you work longer and easier during the day?

If the answer is yes, you have performed a miracle on yourself. You have done what no conventional doctor in the world can do for you. You have stopped your arthritis in its tracks, simply by eliminating certain foods.

And this is just the beginning. If the two week test is successful, you should never again touch those foods, or products made from them as long as you live. Ever. Watch the results.

Perhaps the arthritis will not only be stopped, but actually reversed. As with so many other maladies, if you stop the foods that feed them, you can stop their growth, and begin to starve them It is a simple test. It may be a life-renewing test.

Why not try it — *today!*

The arthritis will not only be stopped, but actually reversed. As with so many other maladies, if you stop the foods that feed them, you can stop their growth.

Diet as a Weapon Against Arthritis

Again, as you've heard a hundred times, overweight is murder to your body. When you overeat, you dig your own grave.

This is especially true for arthritis. The more weight you carry in your flesh, the more pressure you put on your joints. Every ounce hurts! Every ounce you take off takes off that much pressure.

Think of overweight as a corn callous that surrounds your entire body. You let the corn grow too thick, it never stops hurting. But if you take it away, the pressure eases and the pain evaporates.

If you ache, diet that ache away. Forget, for the moment, how you work to achieve your goal. Just concentrate on how much better you'll feel.

Love works miracles but no doctor will prescribe it. You have to give it to yourself, several times a day.

A Little Love Goes a Long Way

If you have arthritis, you are dealing with joints that have been injured by the foods you have unknowingly put into your body, or by a malfunction in your body which you are now going to correct the natural way.

As you know, when you have been injured — emotionally injured, for example, as when somebody insults or snubs you — the one balm you need most is love. You need love when you are hurt, and your joints need love when they are hurt.

Therefore, an absolute requirement of this program for recovery from arthritis is to give your joints the love they need several times a day. This is the simplest healer of them all.

Let's take your fingers, for example. Every few hours at least, take each of your hands and raise it to your lips, and kiss those injured fingers. Feel the kiss on those joints. Feel the love pass through your lips to those brave fingers.

At the same time, say in your mind or through your lips, "I love you. I appreciate how brave you are to give me so much service when you are suffering so much. I'm going to take responsibility now for making you well and young again. I admire you. I love you. I honor your bravery."

This works. It works miracles. Love is stronger than any doctor's drug. But no doctor will prescribe it.

You have to give it to yourself. You have to give it to yourself several times a day.

Never let your joints forget that you love them. That you support them in their struggle. That, no matter how much they have to fight to win, you admire and adore them.

The World's Gentlest Exercises for Arthritis

Almost all arthritis sufferers report morning stiffness and pain. This can, as you know, ruin your entire day, unless you deal with it immediately upon awakening. Since I have arthritis myself, I have studied intensely to overcome this morning stiffness. And now let me pass on to you what I have found.

If you wake up in the morning so stiff that you can't straighten out, why not just roll yourself into a ball. I do. It's simple. It diminishes pain. And it takes only two or three gentle minutes. It's ingenious. It's been my helping angel for years now. Here's how:

Just reach down slowly, and put your hands underneath your knees.

Bring those knees up slowly and gently, as close as you comfortably can to your chest. Rock forward slightly on your curved back. Slowly and gently roll back and forth in bed like a rocking chair, then roll from one side to the other.

This relaxes the muscles in your back and gives them a good, gentle, easy massage.

If you wake up in the morning so stiff that you can't straighten out, roll yourself into a ball. It diminishes pain. And it takes only two or three gentle minutes.

Two Variations

1. Lie on your back in bed or on the floor.

Stretch your arms out to the side at shoulder height.

Gently bring your knees up to your chest.

Slowly and gently roll your body to the left, but turn your head to the right. Keep your shoulders on the floor.

Hold that position while you relax, exhale, and inhale.

Then slowly return to the center.

Roll your body to the right, and your head to the left.

Repeat the sequence four or five times.

2. Lie flat on your back. Bend your knees up, keeping your feet on the floor.

Clasp your hands behind the back of your neck, and gently turn your hips to the left as far as comfortably possible without lifting your shoulders.

Your knees will follow your hips until they approach being flat on the floor.

Hold for a count of ten.

Return to your starting position, and then twist gently to the right.

Repeat four or five times.

Some therapists advise finishing off this gentle exercise by reversing your position. In other words, turn over and lie face down.

Insert your hands between your chest and the mattress or the floor.

Push up, gently lifting your body and making sure to keep your head level with your body rather than your curved back.

Hold for two breaths.

Then slowly lower your body. Repeat two times.

How To Prevent or Loosen Up
A Stiff Neck and Shoulders

If you feel your joints becoming stiff during the day and don't have the opportunity to lie down, here are two easy movements:

1. Sit comfortably or stand, feet about 12 inches apart.

Wrap your arms around your shoulders and drop your head and upper body forward.

Relax into that position, allowing your back to stretch out.

Let your head hang, relaxing the stiff muscles in your neck.

Breathe slowly and deeply five times.

Return to an upright position and relax your arms to your sides.

Repeat whenever you feel the tension building up.

2. Sit, or even comfortably stand. Keep your legs spread a little apart.

Put one hand on your hip, and lean forward from your waist.

Lean only as far as it's comfortable.

Slowly swing your free arm from behind you toward the floor, then up in front of your opposite shoulder.

Have it gently cross your body five times.

Then reverse your arms, and repeat five times.

As you can see, this can be quickly done anytime of the night or day. It not only takes the tightness out of your shoulders, but it also gives your mind a few moments to wander free, and therefore refresh itself.

Words of Caution

❖ Never strain to get more reach when you stretch. In other words, go only as far as comfortable, and not one inch more. You're not out to set records, or attain a "perfect" position. You're simply out to ease the stiffness and pain in your body.

❖ Never hold a position so long that it hurts. Just get the stretch till it begins to feel not so good. And then quit.

❖ And one other caution, if it applies to you. If you have a trainer, check the stretches out with him or her. The more professional opinions you get, the more you benefit, of course.

And if you wish to, I would certainly applaud your asking a physical therapist to run you through the first time you do these or any other stretches. They are professionals, and they can give you the perfect form and timing.

How To Loosen Tight Fingers

The simplest remedy for cramped fingers is to let your hands hang loose, fingers open, and give them a vigorous, repeated shake from the wrist. Visualize them covered with dust and you're shaking them to get that dust off. See the dust falling from your fingers as you shake them.

In a sense this image is absolutely true. The dust is pain and stiffness and you are shaking those away.

This excercise also increases the circulation to your entire arm, so do it several times a day.

Gently massaging and stroking your fingers also helps. Pet, pat and caress them.

You might also gently tighten your fist and hold it for a count of ten. Then release and stretch your hand wide open as far as possible for another count of ten.

Repeat with your other hand and do this throughout the day.

Do Gentle Yoga To Ward Off Arthritis

Yoga exercises, with the calm, thorough stretching they give you, have kept women's joints supple for centuries. Of course, with arthritic knees, you are not going to attempt a full lotus position. And in any event, you should work with a qualified teacher on an individual basis, or in a class small enough to receive personal guidance. . . at least in the beginning.

Here are four of the easiest yoga-based movements. You can slip into them immediately on your own:

1. Gently turn your head to the left, as far as is perfectly comfortable.

Lower it very slowly to your left shoulder, as far as is perfectly comfortable.

Then return it upright to the center and lower it very slowly towards your chest, as far as is comfortable.

Return to the upright position.

Turn it to the right and lower very slowly toward your right shoulder, as far as is comfortable.

Return it to the upright position.

Repeat three times.

If you've taken yoga before, you will recognize this stretch as a modified version of the classic neck roll. But the classic yoga neck roll scrunches vertebrae and therefore is not indicated for arthritic necks. That is why I have so heavily emphasized moving your neck only as far as comfortable. It may be only an inch or two at the beginning. But it will soon grow, and your range of comfort will increase dramatically.

2. Raise your arms over your head.

Clasp your hands and pull them up.

Keeping your hands clasped, lower your left arm and, at the same time, bend your right arm over your head.

Lean towards your left side to get a good stretch.

Then, hands clasped, raise your arms overhead again.

Lower your right arm and, at the same time, bend your left arm over your head.

Lean towards your right side to get a good stretch.

Repeat four times.

3. Stand, or you can sit on a stool.

Clasp your hands behind you.

Keeping your arms straight, raise them as far back as it's comfortable.

At the same time, tilt your head back.

Feel the stretch across your chest and the squeeze in your upper back.

Breathe in and exhale slowly three times.

Relax.

4. Raise your shoulders gently up toward your ears.

Make circles with them from front to back.

Repeat five times.

Then reverse, making circles with your shoulders from back to front five times.

Activities That Bring You Freedom From Pain

Lucky you, if you have a swimming pool, lake or ocean nearby because swimming is the best overall form of exercise, particularly for someone who is in pain. The water supports your body weight so you are free to move without the pull of gravity — and with less pain.

Can't get to a "swimming hole" or you're afraid of deep water? Then try your bathtub or shower! Warm water (not hot or cold) is very conducive to relaxing tight muscles and relieving stress in the body. Sore joints and muscles seem to feel less pain in water.

Bicycling is a great way to exercise the joints and muscles. If you are in too much pain to go for a ride, try a stationary bike and pedal at a comfortable speed, increasing it as you build up your stamina. Eventually, you will realize a stronger body with less pain.

Go dancing! Music has a hypnotic way of making you forget your pain. Dance with a partner or go solo. Through the movement of your body to the tempo, you will be lubricating all your joints in an enjoyable way.

Walking is the simplest form of exercise. Take a long walk, always moving a little faster than you normally do. Breathe deeply as you go briskly down the road. Swing your arms in rhythm with your feet. This will activate your upper body circulation.

Note: I prefer fast walking to running. It is just as effective and does not shock the body joints. I also carry a cassette player with earphones so I can walk in rhythm to the music. You'll be amazed at how far you can go in a very short time. Remember, you have to return so time your walk. If you plan to walk for 20 minutes, go 10 minutes in one direction, then turn around and walk the 10 minutes back to your starting point. How good you will feel when your body is functioning on all cylinders.

So, "put a little fun in your life" and reap the benefits of your activities!

Relieving Stress

Stress is one of the factors contibuting to the pain of arthritis. It causes the muscles to tense up, the blood vessels to constrict and the toxins to build up in your body. Before you realize it, you are "tied up in knots."

Relaxation is the only way to undo these effects of stress. One of my favorite ways of getting rid of that pain is to take a trip to a tropical island. The warm, moist air soothes my aching muscles.

I lie on the beach . . . listen to the ocean waves breaking on the shore . . . look up at a clear blue sky with billowy white clouds . . . watch a fiery sunset . . . listen to romantic music in the moonlight.

So what if it is only a temporary escape from the reality of your everyday routine. You are giving your body and mind a chance to recuperate and soothe your frazzled nerves. The chemistry in your body has a chance to clear the toxins away.

How quickly my pain goes away when I am being good to myself!

If you are not able to get away, try meditation in a quiet place. Let your mind soar to a place of tranquility. Bring peace and quiet to your mind and body.

Biofeedback training is very helpful in recognizing your pattern of stress in the body. It will help you see when you are being affected by stress stimulants. When you are aware of a stress-producing situation at the outset, you can counteract its progress.

Relaxation has been proven to lessen, even remove, the pain.

Massage is another enjoyable way to relax and ease the pain. Have your mate or a friend do the honors, or go to a professional. You can also do spot massaging yourself. Try using a mentholated oil or any over-the-counter preparation for arthritis sufferers and slowly rub your painful joints. You will be amazed at the relief you can give yourself.

Passivity Gets You Nowhere

Arthritis, of course, comes in many forms. Therefore, some of the specific techniques and exercises I've described may not be right for you, but the underlying principle still applies.

These simple, gentle stretches relieve creaky joints and toning the muscle around those joints takes that horrible, continuous, unremitting pressure off.

And, my dietary suggestions are helpful for anyone, even if you don't have arthritis.

The point is to take as active a role as you can in combating the onset and symptoms of this disease.

You'll be amazed at the difference it makes!

SUMMARY

Physical Treatments

- bicycling
- capsaicin ointment (derived from cayenne, chili peppers, jalapenos, paprika, red peppers)
- creams made for arthritis sufferers
- dancing
- exercises
- heat treatment gloves for arthritic hands
- jacuzzi baths
- massages
- neck roll when sleeping
- proper sitting and standing postures
- reflexology
- relaxation
- soft cervical collar when sleeping
- soft chiropractic adjustments
- stretches
- swimming
- trager

Nutritional Aids

- boswellia
- cod liver oil
- evening primrose oil
- fish: cod, herring, mackerel, salmon, swordfish
- fo-ti
- ginger
- guggul
- ho-shou-wu
- omega-3 oil
- rohitukine
- selenium
- vitamin B-complex
- vitamin E
- vitamin C
- vitamin B^6
- warm fluids
- yucca

Zinc

- egg yolks
- herring
- liver
- peanut butter
- sesame seeds
- soy products
- sunflower seeds
- whole grains

Copper

- avocados
- chocolate
- dried peas and beans
- nuts
- organ meats
- prunes
- raisins
- seafood

Caution! Avoid!

- eggplant
- ice cream
- red and green peppers
  (internally)
- soft drinks
- sweets
- tobacco
- tomatoes
- white flour
- white potatoes
- white sugar

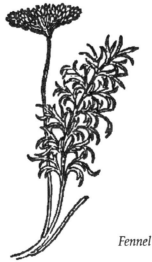

Fennel

7

Asthma: How To Stop the Wheeze

*I*n all the world, there is nothing more frightening than asthma. I have several friends who suffer from it, and my heart pours out to them whenever I see them with an attack . . . or even when I hear their heavy breathing on the phone.

If you have asthma, you depend on your inhaler, and it is an excellent medical tool, giving great relief without known side effects. So far, so good.

But the same certainly cannot be said for the various pills that may also be prescribed for you. As the medical record proves only too well, some do actually aggravate your condition, depending, of course, upon your individual case. And steroids such as prednisone are notorious for thinning bones.

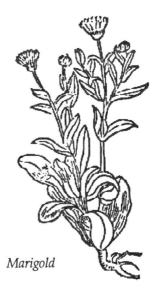

Marigold

81

Are You Getting Your "Asthma Vitamins" Today?

The alternative medicine of natural healing has proven, again and again, that pills and expensive inhalers are not the only solution. Why rely on them entirely, or perhaps even at all, when there are so many natural ways to take control of your asthma?

❖ For example, do you know the effect of inexpensive vitamins on your asthma?

❖ Do you know which hot drinks calm asthma?

❖ Do you know about the effect of onions on the disease?

❖ Have you tried chili peppers?

❖ Other ways to cope range from simply remembering to wear a scarf and muffle your nose and mouth in cold weather to doing gentle aerobics.

Any one, or combination of these methods has been proved to alleviate asthma to a surprising degree.

This chapter will tell you how to conquer asthma and have a young woman's lungs again.

Vitamin B^6 and C

> **Foods rich in vitamin B^6 include: Brewer's yeast, brown rice, hazelnuts, sunflower seeds, lentils, rye, whole wheat and soybeans.**

The most recent studies indicate that vitamin B^6 is highly beneficial. For example, Dr. Robert Reynolds, a United States Department of Agriculture biochemist, concludes that many asthmatics need more of this vitamin than usual, because of a genetic error in their metabolism.

You should take between 50-100 mg of vitamin B^6 supplements daily. The results will not be apparent at first, but they will often kick in a month or so later.

Many asthmatics also have a low level of vitamin C. Let's look at the *National Health and Nutrition Examination Survey* of 9,100 adults which revealed that:

"Above average intake of vitamin C — 200 milligrams more than the 98 milligram average — was associated with about a 30 percent lower incidence of bronchitis and wheezing."

This conclusion was backed up by Nobel winner Dr. Linus Pauling and by tests done at Yale University, in Nigeria and in South Africa. Based on the results of these tests, daily doses of 500 to 1,000 mg of vitamin C may actually conquer asthma.

How? By reducing your sensitivity to the irritants in the air that often provoke such attacks.

You should eat many of the foods rich in vitamin C. These include:

Brussels sprouts, broccoli, cabbage, cantaloupe, cherries, chives, citrus fruit, collard greens, green peppers, mangoes, mustard greens, papaya, parsley, rose hips, strawberries, tomatoes and watercress.

"Above average intake of Vitamin C – 200 mg more than the 98 mg average – was associated with about a 30 percent lower incidence of bronchitis and wheezing."

Are Food Poisons — Food Allergies — Causing Your Asthma Attacks?

Studies from all over the world — from Minnesota to Israel — indicate that dairy products trigger asthma attacks in many women. Why not try a 14-day dairy elimination diet to see if it relieves your problem.

When you get rid of the dairy foods, remember this. Not only do milk and cheese products have to go, but also all milk included in the processed foods you buy. Read the labels carefully. And protect your lungs.

Then there's what is called the "Chinese restaurant syndrome." These are actually bad asthma allergy reactions to monosodium glutamate (MSG), which was once used in almost every Chinese restaurant you went into.

Fortunately, the Chinese are one of the smartest people on earth, and many now prepare their foods without MSG. Always ask when you're in one of their restaurants whether you can get your favorite dish free of this little poisoner. The flavor will be as good, but the attack may be thwarted.

Also, be aware that packaged foods may contain MSG as well. Always, but always, carefully read the label first on everything you buy.

There is another common offender, sulfite, a preservative used for generations in wine and beer making. Sulfites are also used in food processing to stop the browning due to oxidation. Some grocers and salad bar operators add sulfites to their produce to keep it looking fresh when it is not. If you have ever felt wheezy after salad bar fare, sulfites may be the culprit. Ask whether they are being used. Speak up. Protect your lungs.

Also, if you are sulfite sensitive, remember that the preservative is often present in dried fruit.

Additionally, nuts, salt and some seafoods also affect most asthmatics.

And then there is the yellow food dye, tartrazine (F, D and C yellow dye #5). This is used in one processed food after another and can bring on rather violent asthma attacks. Again, read the labels.

How To Rebuild Your Tortured Lungs and Airways

Every single day, you should eat rose hips, berries, and the rind and pulp (including the white part) of citrus fruit. Let me repeat that: you should not only eat the fruit of the citrus, but also its pulp and rind.

Why? Because all these natural nourishers not only contain vitamin C, which you have already seen alleviates asthma, but they also offer you the extra booster of bioflavonoid enzymes.

What are these? They are natural "repair enzymes" that restore the delicate alveoli and capillaries in your fragile lungs and airways, and protect them from the irritating substances you may be inhaling.

Let me repeat this again. Rose hips, most berries, and the rind and pulp of citrus fruits not only protect you against future asthma attacks, but actually repair your lungs and airways. They rebuild your lungs and airways. They bring you back, day after day, towards normality. They therefore can be thought of as reversing asthma, making you better and better, and going further and further away from it.

So, to get the full benefit from citrus foods, eat them whole. What does this mean? Remove the skin gently, then eat as much of the white part around the

Rose hips, berries, and the rind and pulp of citrus fruits not only protect you against future asthma attacks, but actually repair your lungs and airways. They bring you back to normality. Think of them as reversing asthma, making you better and better . . .

pulp in oranges, tangerines, and even grapefruit, as possible.

Make every orange you eat into an orange sandwich. Think of the rind as two slices of delicious enzyme bread, surrounding the fruit underneath. Chomp away on as much as you want of it.

Remember, with every bite of it, you are one step further away from those weak lungs.

Grapes also have large amounts of these bioflavonoid enzymes and therefore should always be eaten with their skins. Forget Mae West, with her famous line: "Peel me a grape."

Some Like It Hot — Even If They're Asthmatic

Chili pepper (capsicum) is an old home remedy for cutting phlegm and clearing your airways. It has been doing it for centuries. And now modern medical research validates its effectiveness.

For example, pulmonary expert Dr. Irwin Ziment calls chili pepper "nature's *Robitussin*," and often prescribes it for his patients. He notes that sometimes the effect can be profound. Apparently, the initial, fiery sensation in your mouth sets off a dramatic reaction in your bronchial tubes and lungs that dilutes the sticky accumulations blocking them.

By clearing out these sticky accumulations, these hot peppers automatically facilitate your breathing. It becomes easier and more natural and you have that wonderful feeling of more breath entering your lungs as the pain drains out of them.

Think of it. When you are stuffed up with a cold and you eat foods spiced with a hot pepper, not only does your pallet tingle, but your nasal and sinus passages clear like magic as well.

No pills or prescriptions are involved, of course. Just natural, readily available, inexpensive spices.

The exact same magic works on your asthma!

So sprinkle red pepper flakes on your pizza. Make garlic, oil or red pepper sauce for spaghetti, or go for Tex-Mex and curries!

Cayenne pepper, jalapenos, or most bottled hot sauces, such as the classic Tabasco sauce, are other good sources of capsicum.

Drinks That Soothe Asthma

Recent Canadian studies and Pennsylvania allergist and immunologist Mark Shamplain, M.D. concur about coffee. The charge of caffeine it contains — besides being a proven pick-me-up — is a well-known bronchodilator.

Caffeine is also chemically related to theophylline, a drug often prescribed for asthmatics. However, some patients find this drug far too strong. So why not try a few cups of coffee a day instead — but no more than three, please — to give you relief without side effects.

Also, there is mullein tea, the ancient natural antidote for asthma dating back to the Greek physician Dioscorides. With this brew, you may prefer to inhale its steam rather than drink it. It is a member of the figwort family, and in dry form it can be "gathered" in health food stores. Its effectiveness as demulcent and expectorant derives from a concentration of mucilage in the plant.

Never, but never, use aluminum. First, aluminum can react detrimentally with herbs, leaching out their power. Second, *it can kill your brain cells!* Please throw out *any* aluminum pot or container.

In other words, it not only soothes and protects your poor, irritated mucous membranes, but it also enables you to spit up the harsh chemicals that are irritating them.

Use a ceramic, glass or stainless steel utensil to make mullein or any herbal tea. Never, but never, use aluminum. First, aluminum can react detrimentally with herbs, leaching out their power. And second, it can kill your brain cells.

Please throw out any aluminum pot or container you have in the house.

Ease the Wheeze with Onion and Honey

This is another time-proven remedy for asthma and bronchitis. What you do is eat slices of raw onion or inhale its fumes while slicing it. Yes, it makes your eyes tear, but it also clears out those clogged airways.

Or, you might try eating honey which was the ancient Greek remedy. They probably felt that ingesting the traces of pollen found in honey could desensitize you to such pollen. In other words, it worked much the same way pollen shots do if you are allergic to pollen.

Better still, you can combine the two, in these two ways:

❖ Put onions in a blender, mix the extract with honey, add lemon juice. Blend well. Eat a teaspoonful three to four times a day.

❖ Or if you prefer– put thin slices of onions on a plate and convert them to a honey and onion sandwich by covering them over with honey and letting them sit overnight. Then, scrape off the honey and eat a teaspoonful of it three to four times a day.

Allow Time For Your Food To Digest!

Be sure to allow at least 3-4 hours between your last meal and bedtime, so your food has a chance to digest before you lie down. Going to bed on a full stomach is a good way to invite heartburn, indigestion, obesity, and the possibility of another asthma attack which can be brought on by escaping acid from a stomach reflux. If you find it impossible to stay awake and active after eating, be sure to prop yourself up in bed and take anantacid to reduce the acid produced in your stomach.

Fish Oil Comes to the Rescue Again

There is great new hope on the horizon for asthmatics. The most recent research suggests that asthma may be an inflammatory disease in which inflammatory chemicals called leukotrienes run wild and cause constriction of your bronchial tubes.

Why do these tubes constrict? Because the inflamation swells them and restricts their passages. This sounds pretty much like arthritis, where the joints also swell. So natural healing doctors have responded to this common sense resemblance, and prescribed fish oil—EPA's or Omega-3 oils—to their patients. It blocks the leukotrienes just as it blocks the inflammatory agents around the arthritic joints.

Therefore, in proven, documented case after case, it has brought surprising relief.

Why not try it for yourself, tomorrow?

Natural healing doctors prescribe fish oil – EPA's or Omega-3 oils. In proven, documented case after case, it has brought surprising relief.

Possible Allergens To Avoid

If you first developed asthma in your middle years, then this section is of utmost importance to you. Asthma that strikes late in life could be caused by a buildup, over the years, of sensitivity to allergens in your environment or your food that your body simply sloughed off when you were younger.

If this is true, you want to find out about it immediately. But it can cost weeks and a small fortune to take a full set of allergy tests. So you really should do it for yourself, in this way:

Keep an asthma diary. Every day, enter into it when your seizures take place, and whether they seem to follow a pattern of exposure to food or a prevailing indoor/outdoor condition.

In order to do this accurately, this diary, at least in the beginning, must contain all your daily meals and snacks — everything you eat during the day. And it must contain the daily weather conditions you encounter.

In this way, when a seizure strikes, you can simply look back in your diary and see what foods or conditions might have caused or contributed to it.

For instance, there is a polyunsaturated fatty acid called PUFA. It is found in vegetables and such nut oils as corn, peanut, safflower, sunflower and walnut, among others. Nutritional experts now feel it may be a hidden contributor to asthma seizures, so keep special track of foods that contain it.

If you use a lot of oil in cooking or salad dressing, consider substituting vegetable oil.

No Smoking

If you smoke, stop. Stop now. Stop for good.

If you do not smoke, avoid smoke-filled rooms. This is harder, but with a little sense of self-preservation, it certainly can be done.

Tobacco smoke is a prime irritant to your airways, as is any smoke. Therefore, unfortunately, cozy evenings in front of the fireplace, or heating your country retreat with wood burning stoves may also be out of the question. Wood smoke just does not agree with most asthmatics.

Mentholated Sauna

Warm, humid air makes breathing much easier. If you don't have access to a mentholated sauna, there are a few ways to create one at home. Put a humidifier in the room where you sleep. Try a little eucalyptus in your cold or hot water humidifier.

Make a mentholated steambath by putting some eucalyptus oil in boiling water and placing the steaming pot in your bathroom. The warm moisture from your bathtub or shower will pick up the scent and spread it to your nostrils.

You can get a more direct effect by placing your head over a pot of warm/hot water with eucalyptus oil in it. Put a towel over your head to prevent the steam from escaping, but test the temperature of the steam before you put your face into it so you won't burn yourself.

Caution: Air passages do not like very hot or very cold temperatures, so keep the water warm.

Other Frequent Allergens

Never treat
yourself like
an invalid
just because
you have
asthma.
Many
athletes
have the
condition,
including
olympic stars.

Here are the common allergens for asthmatics:

Hair sprays, perfumes, cleaning fluids, paint fumes, insecticides, house dust, dander from pets, gasoline or car exhaust fumes, pollens and molds.

Most can be avoided, or certainly cut down. For example, if pollen seems to touch off seizures, remain indoors as much as possible, with the windows closed during those seasons when pollen and mold spore counts are the highest.

If you have to go out driving, don't run your air-conditioning on the setting that brings in outside air.

Exercises for Asthmatics

Never, never treat yourself like an invalid just because you have asthma. Always remember, many athletes have or have had the condition . . . including olympic stars.

According to Francois Haas, Director of Pulmonary Rehabilitation Training in New York University's Rusk Center, regular aerobic exercise is not harmful. It is helpful. Quite helpful.

At the Rusk Center, patients are carefully monitored while using treadmills, stationary bicycles, rowing and cross-country skiing machines. These monitors prove that the exercise immensely benefits their asthma. They are then encouraged to continue on their own, mostly with home equipment, but also by doing the real thing.

Of course, walking, cycling, etc. three or four times a week is usually beneficial. Of great help.

Talk to your physician about an exercise program. But, at the very least, learn and practice deep breathing techniques such as the ones below. These will enable you to increase the amount of oxygen you can bring into your lungs. And they will help those poor lungs get out the stale air that irritates them.

Do the Cobra

This yoga posture aids asthmatics greatly by opening the breathing passages. Here is how you do it:

❖ Lie on your stomach, with your arms at your sides. Inhale as deeply as you can and raise your head and trunk. Slide your arms forward, placing your hands palm down for support. Hold this position by straightening your arms as much as is comfortable.

❖ Exhale as deeply as you can. While you are exhaling, make the same hissing sound as a cobra.

❖ Then, when the air has completely left your lungs, slowly lower yourself to the floor. Relax for a count of five. Repeat the exercise at least five times.

Relax and Live Longer!

You will breathe easier, too. Tension and stress cause your muscles to tighten and your breathing to become shallow.

Do yourself a favor by taking a muscle tension check every now and then. Are your shoulders riding high? Are you filling your lungs with each breath? Are the muscles in your face tense? Is your jaw closed tightly?

Do yourself a favor by taking a muscle tension check. Are your shoulders riding high? Are you filling your lungs with each breath?

Exercises that expand your lung capacity are wonderful for bringing tranquility to your body. The action of deep breathing will slow down your panic triggers and release the stress that constricts your air passages.

Take a deep breath and let your shoulders fall in a relaxed slump. Let your head fall to your chest. Slowly lower your head and upper body toward the floor and just hang loose. Breathe in and out as you let all the tension flow through your fingertips toward the floor. Pretend you are a rag doll and let your arms and hands flop around as you gently bounce from the waist. Now, slowly roll your body up, one vertebra at a time. Let your head be the last thing to come up.

You should feel rejuvenated with a relaxed energy.

Always carry your chest high with your shoulders relaxed. This will free your diaphragm to work your lungs.

Life is so much more enjoyable when you can breathe easily and relax.

SUMMARY

Foods and Vitamins That Help:

Vitamin B^6

- brewer's yeast
- brown rice
- hazelnuts
- lentils
- rye
- soybeans
- sunflower seeds
- whole wheat

Vitamin C

- broccoli
- brussels sprouts
- cabbage
- cantaloupe
- cherries
- chives
- citrus fruits & rinds
- collard greens
- grapes
- green peppers
- mangoes
- mustard greens
- papayas
- parsley
- rose hips
- strawberries
- tomatoes
- watercress

Also Have

- caffeine
- cayenne pepper
- chili pepper
- curries
- fish (omega-3 oils)
- honey
- jalapenos
- lemons
- mullein tea
- onions
- tabasco sauce

Try

- aerobic exercises
- baths
- bicycles
- cross-country skiing machines
- deep breathing exercises
- eucalyptus saunas
- fast walking
- humifidiers
- rowing
- showers
- treadmills
- yoga

Foods and Preservatives To Avoid

- corn oil
- dairy products
- dried fruits
- F, D and C
  yellow dye #5
- monosodium
  glutamate (msg)
- nuts
- peanut oil
- safflower oil
- salt
- seafood
- sulfites
- sunflower oil
- walnuts

Also Avoid

- cleaning fluids
- dander from pets
- exhaust fumes
- gasoline fumes
- hair sprays
- house dust
- insecticides
- molds
- paint fumes
- perfumes
- pollens
- tobacco smoke and
  wood smoke
- very hot or very cold
  temperatures

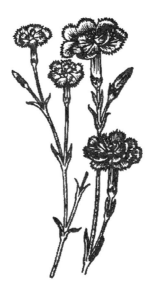

8

Cholesterol: How To Have A Young Woman's Cholesterol As Long As You Live

$\mathcal{L}$et me make two assumptions at the very beginning of this chapter.

The first is that you already know approximately how "high" your cholesterol is today.

The second is that you think it is much, much too high, that you are worried about it, and that you fervently seek new ways to keep it from going higher, and want to bring it back to what you consider a "normal" range.

Fine. So I don't have to define "cholesterol" for you. Nor do I have to pass on to you the usual scientific jargon about what causes it, what different kinds there are, etc., etc.

Let me put it to you as simply as this. Cholesterol is good for you up to a certain point. And, from that point on, it is bad for you.

We all know this, of course. Everyone seems to be talking about nothing else these days. So much emphasis has been put on cholesterol that knowing your serum level has almost

If we
monitor
our
cholesterol
to help
us gauge
our future
health and
longevity,
we can
live our
lives
delightfully
and sanely,
remaining
in
Second
Youth
until
80, 90, 100
and even
120
youthful
years
of age.

become like knowing your height and weight.

Why? Because it is a vital statistic telling you about the future, strength and endurance of your heart.

But researchers have recently found that it is only *one* of such statistics. You must understand this deeply. Your cholesterol level, by itself, does not and cannot predict heart attacks. It does not and cannot, by itself, predict narrowing arteries, heart pain, varicose veins, shortness of breath, heart palpitations, and the flood of other coronary symptoms we all live in dread of daily.

Cholesterol level is only one of the many measurements we use to gauge our future health and longevity. It is important, but not sufficient by itself to either damage or destroy us. And, if we use the cholesterol measurement to help us live our life delightfully and sanely, it can keep us in Second Youth until 80, 90, 100 or even 120 youthful years of age.

Let's Set Up a Second-Youth Cholesterol Goal For Ourselves

Of course, I would like to see you have a cholesterol serum level of 180 or 200, and so would every doctor I know. But those figures entail almost daily drudgery, deprivation and fasting, and I don't feel that any life-loving woman can stay on that rigid a diet for very long.

So I have chosen for myself, and I recommend to you, a serum cholesterol level of approximately 220. That's about halfway between the level that your sternest doctor wants, and the real danger level of 240.

So you're going to aim for 220. But you're going to aim for it in the context of good eating . . . a happy life . . . a life full of the exercises and stretches I give you elsewhere in this book . . . and the kind of non-worried relaxation that allows you to cheat with a banana split every so often.

I call my way, "joyful cholesterol lowering" and then, "joyful cholesterol maintenance." You have fun, and darn good meals, getting it down to the proper figure of 220. And you have even more fun keeping it there for the rest of your Second Youth.

I call my way "joyful cholesterol lowering" and then "joyful cholesterol maintenance." You have fun keeping it that way for the rest of your Second Youth.

Good Cholesterol *vs.* Bad Cholesterol

There is often a lot of talk about "good" high-density lipoproteins (HDL) and artery-clogging, low-density cholesterol (LDL). These are also essential to your calculations and to your dieting fun, but let's just throw out the highfaluting words, and call them good cholesterol and bad cholesterol.

I was completely dismayed when my cholesterol test showed my count to be above normal. My doctor calmed me down by explaining that the ratio between the HDL and the LDL counts put me in the safe zone. However, he encouraged me to watch my diet and lower the count, just to prevent going over the limit.

My suggestion, if you are worried about your cholesterol, is to ask your doctor to explain what your LDL/HDL cholesterol ratio is, get his advice, and then follow it.

Foods That Cut Total Cholesterol And Raise the Amount of Good Cholesterol

These, above all, are olive oil and onions. Use olive oil on your salads every single day. Use onions in your meals at least every other day (include parsley after the meal to kill the odor).

These two steps alone have solved many cholesterol problems, and they are just yummy.

Next are apples — delicious. Beans of all kinds. Also delicious, but don't forget the *Beano* if they give you gas. Then green plantains and yogurt. Also delicious.

So now you're fighting cholesterol with one treat after another. But here's perhaps the most surprising one of all. Recent research has also found that the moderate use of alcohol — and that means no more than one or two drinks per day — also raises the good cholesterol in your blood. So don't be guilty in the slightest when you have your evening cocktail, but also don't imbibe if you shouldn't medically, or if you have other reasons not to.

And finally there is green tea. One cup a day is the prescription. It has the same effect as two drinks, or can be used to supplement their good-cholesterol building powers.

Now Let's Look at the Grains and Vegetables That Lower Artery-Clogging Bad Cholesterol

The most famous of these is, of course, oat bran. There's no doubt that it is terrific in the morning, but only in moderate portions, please. Also, should you feel that it tastes rather like ground-up shirt cardboard, rest assured that whole wheat or barley are just as remedial.

The cholesterol-lowering vegetables range from artichokes, beets, carrots and eggplant to reishi or shiitake mushrooms and spinach. Include them in every lunch or dinner.

And, if you just can't stay away from fatty foods, don't hate yourself. Instead, recent findings at the University of Texas show that eggplant, in particular, stops the rise of serum-cholesterol level when these fatty foods are consumed.

Then there's garlic. If you like it, eat it straight. If not, take capsules of liquid garlic extract. Researchers in India, France and California have proved its benefits.

Researchers in Thailand have produced good results with chili pepper — and there is also ginger, seaweed and seafood.

So there's absolutely no shortage of bad cholesterol lowering foods.

Forget about expensive medical drugs with their dangerous side effects.

Sweep out the cholesterol by stuffing yourself with good food instead.

Fruits That Fight Cholesterol . . . and Win!

Again, an apple a day. Then there are the ever-reliable friends, citrus fruits. Grapefruit seems to be the most healing of all of them, due to super-powerful compounds contained in its pectin. And remember, when you eat a grapefruit, the white part of it is equally as healthy as the fruit itself, so eat that too.

Or, if grapefruit doesn't appeal to you, the gelatinous pectin can be taken in supplement form.

Then there's lemon and lime which both have super-high concentrates of acid-based enzymes. These help liquefy the fats that have just entered your body because they combine chemically with them and flush them right out of your body.

Here's an excellent cholesterol-slashing strategy. It comes from the Italians who are among the world's greatest chefs. Serve a slice or two of lemon with beefsteak, veal chops, or cutlets. Squeeze lemon juice on the meat before you eat a single bite, using it in place of salt. It not only enhances the flavor, but it slashes the fat absorption that can take place inside your body.

In other words, it's almost as though you never eat the fat at all as far as your bloodstream, your arteries, and your heart are concerned.

Other fruits proven to drive your cholesterol level down include blackberries, blueberries and strawberries, as well as pineapple and papaya. Papaya, especially, is loaded with the fat-splitting enzyme called papain.

If It Swims or Flies, It Will Carry You To Second Youth at 120

Fish and chicken. The two great cholesterol conquerors. What new information can I tell you about them? First, let me affirm and confirm what every other healer has said — *they are the best!* They give you the protein you need. The substance you need. The energy you need. The bulk in your stomach you need. The feeling of being full and satisfied you need. The chewability you need. The flavor and satisfaction you most desperately need.

I personally love fowl. You, on the other hand, may love fish. Both are excellent, though they work a little differently. In fowl, you take off the skin and the fat that comes underneath it. In fish — especially salmon, etc. — you eat the skin because it contains the Omega-3 fatty acids that protect you against heart disease.

However, I am a chicken skin addict, and I sometimes almost weep when I peel all that delicious skin off my favorite chicken thigh. So I've adopted the one-for-three plan. It's as simple as this: in one meal of fowl out of every three, I simply eat the bird with the skin on.

This is also because we do need fat, and we do need cholesterol . . . just not too much of either.

Fat is a plumping and beauty food. It keeps the skin of our face and body supported with a cushioned foundation, instead of thinning it to the point of appearing gaunt. And it helps skin retain its smoothness and healthy young color. That's why people on crash diets look so much like concentration camp prisoners.

So, one meal out of every three with poultry, eat the skin too. Have a ball. Let go here and you won't be tempted to let go there, in your favorite dessert shop.

Here is the paramount rule: *Don't* serve the same kind of fish or fowl over and over again, to the point of terminal boredom. Try different recipes: Southern, Middle Eastern, Thai, Spanish, Barbecued, etc. Have Cornish hen, duck, goose, pheasant or turkey, every so often.

Turkey, especially, should be eaten by all of us far more often than it is. Its white meat has the lowest fat and cholesterol count of any fowl. And it has bulk, it's delicious, it satisfies your taste buds and the hollow of your stomach. You can never overindulge. Eat. Enjoy.

Buy turkey parts at your butcher. Don't forget, have one meal out of three with the skin left on. Satisfy your craving for fats; just don't let them drown you.

The best fish are the cold and/or saltwater kind. They include bluefish, herring, mackerel, salmon, sardines, and tuna. Once we thought they were no-no's, because they are high in polyunsaturated fat, but now they are widely recommended in almost every medical report you can read. This is because they are rich in the Omega-3 fatty acids that serve as your shield against heart disease and heart attacks.

Incidentally, another great source of Omega-3 fatty acids is sunflower seeds or even canola oil. Both are options you should consider for cooking and for salad dressing.

A Nutty and Very Smart Way
To Slash Cholesterol

There is a brand-new study published in the prestigious *New England Journal of Medicine* that says regular consumption of nuts reduces your cholesterol levels.

Let's look at the facts. Volunteers were put on two carefully controlled diets for two months. One was a nut-free, standard low-cholesterol diet. The other was exactly the same, except that 20 percent of its calories came from walnuts.

While all the volunteers in both studies benefited, the nut eaters' cholesterol declined an additional 12 percent.

Think of it. If your cholesterol level is 250 today, cutting it an additional 12 percent is slashing off another 30 points, just by eating walnuts — the delicious, nutritious way to say goodbye to 30 points of cholesterol.

But, remember, they are high in calories. So substitute them for some of the other fattening foods you ordinarily eat, such as chocolate ice cream, a hamburger, etc.

Once Again, Nature Trounces
The Huge Pharmaceutical Companies

Another test has shown that guggul, also called gum guggul, is equal to, or better than a standard cholesterol-lowering drug such as *Clofibrate*. Goodbye dangerous drugs! Hello nature's own healers! Go to your health food store, buy a bottle there, and follow the instructions.

And, another astounding recent finding. In a Finnish study, women who took 1/4 ounce of activated charcoal three times a day for four weeks had an overall drop of 40 percent in bad cholesterol. Think of it! A 40 percent drop in four weeks. You can get it for very little at your neighborhood health store.

Let the Cleansing Get Deeper, And Deeper, and Deeper

So you see, we have a vast amount of delicious cholesterol-cleansers to choose from. How, then, do you choose among them? And how many should you eat every day?

The most effective answer is also the simplest. If you have a favorite — such as grapefruit — binge on it. Eat it, white and pulp and all, for breakfast, dinner, and before bed. Indulge. Stuff yourself with it. Eat it until it comes out of your ears.

But, most probably, you will wind up discovering four or five of these cholesterol-cleansers that you continually enjoy. In that case, simply vary your meals every day with one or the other of them. See if you can eat even two or three of them a day. Snack on them. It's like taking out a brand new insurance policy on your heart every single day.

Through eating cholesterol-cleansers, the good cholesterol soars and soars, and the bad cholesterol dips and dips. You're washing age right out of your arteries. You're building Second Youth into every molecule of your body.

By doing this, you're building a cumulative effect. The good cholesterol soars and soars, and the bad cholesterol dips and dips. Every single day, your vital arteries become cleaner and cleaner. You're washing age right out of them. You're building Second Youth into every molecule of your body.

With this much variety to choose from, it's almost impossible to become bored. This is what I have basically discovered — that there's absolutely no reason for you to *fast* your way to great health when it's far easier to *feast* your way instead.

Concentrated Cholesterol Dissolvers

Are You Getting Enough Vitamin C?

Among this vitamin's many preventive and healing properties is lowering your cholesterol level. Why? Because vitamin C is the concentrated healing secret of so many fruits and vegetables. And many of them are simply not in season every month of the year. So why not take a supplement of at least 500 mg a day, and preferably 1000 mg a day, every day? There is an extra bonus to boot: vitamin C prevents hardening of your arteries by preventing the snags and crags and cracks in them that permit cholesterol build-up.

Are You Getting Your Vitamin E?

Sometimes it is difficult to get this priceless vitamin from your food. Therefore, take 400 to 800 mg a day in supplement form. This amount has been shown to improve cholesterol burn-up by your body, and also lower the tendency of the platelets in your arteries to clump together. A double benefit, all through one little pill.

Are You Getting Your Niacin?

In the experience of such practitioners as Dr. Edwin Boyle, niacin (vitamin B^3) not only lowers cholesterol levels, but it also eliminates sludging, the bunching up of red blood cells that clog the blood supply to your heart. In Dr. Boyle's opinion, people who have too high a cholesterol level, as well as any kind of vascular disease, do as well with niacin as with any other regime.

Of course, in Dr. Boyle's test he found that the niacin supplementation must be followed by proper diet and moderate exercise. But isn't this what you are doing with this book right now, every day? One caution however: before you take niacin, consult a good, nutritionally-oriented doctor. Get his recommendation on dosage, and take it along with your B-Complex to get the fullest benefits.

Now, What Foods Do You Have To Cut Back On, And How Much?

We all know that such a cholesterol-cutting regime comes with a big *must* — cutting back on cholesterol-containing foods. The United States Department of Agriculture, the Surgeon General, and the American Heart Association recommend limiting *all* fat consumption — saturates, monosaturates and polysaturates — to no more than 30 percent of all the calories you consume every day.

All fats, however, are not the same. The principal artery-clogger is saturated fat. Its excess consumption is the major cause of high cholesterol levels — three times worse than that of other foods high in dietary cholesterol. In other words, meat, including innards, and most dairy are the most threatening, while eggs — believe it or not — are not nearly that grievous.

In fact, the American Heart Association now allows four eggs a week instead of three. But I think that if you follow the other rules in this book, you can easily and safely stretch that to six.

My late husband, who was a surgeon, was a staunch believer in red meat as the best source of complete protein. He did not want to operate on people who did not eat it because he was convinced they did not heal as well. He was immensely bright, extremely competent as a doctor, and I still follow his point of view by having lean red meat at least once a week.

Here is how I solved the whole problem of what foods to cut down on.

I simply eat less of anything grown on the hoof, whether choice or cheap. This means that two or three servings a week are enough. The rest of my protein I gain from fish and fowl.

I also cut out processed foods, such as liverwurst, cold cuts, hot dogs, patés, sausages and bacon. Or, to be perfectly frank, I cut them out *most* of the time. Once every month or so, when the old habits overwhelm me once again, I do indulge. My theory is to *not* be unforgivingly strict, but to allow a once-in-a-while treat for yourself. That usually prevents a rebellious binge.

As for dairy products, I really don't like the low-fat versions, because they are simply flavorless to me. Therefore, what I do is have what I really like, but in moderation. In other words, it is better for me to have a great piece of cheese once or twice a week, rather than some bland, artificial version every day.

Moderation simply means "every so often." If you used to have a chocolate milk shake every day, make it every week now. Don't put butter on your bread with every meal, but just have it on your breakfast toast, for example. Save the franks for the ball games, and serve barbecued fish for your summer outings.

The Only No-No's

The only things you must eliminate completely are tropical oils, the palm and coconut oils. No, you don't cook with them every day. In fact, it's possible you don't use them in your cooking at all. So much the better.

But they are — without a doubt — rampant on your supermarket shelves. Look at every package you buy, every one of the packaged cereals, bakery goods, non-dairy creamers, and other processed foods that you buy.

For heaven's sake, don't be taken in by labels or stickers advertising "no cholesterol." That is sheer bunk. The plant foods in those packages — grains, legumes, vegetables and fruits — have never contained cholesterol, and never will. *But what else is in the package?*

Read every word on the label. Look for the words *palm oil. . . coconut oil. . . partially hydrogenated.*

If any one of them appear anywhere on that label, even at the end of the list, toss that package away as though it were poison, because it is.

One Final Word: Cholesterol Test Results Are Not Always Accurate

The results on any cholesterol test are only as good as the laboratory that runs it. Therefore, if the results from your test are scary, have them immediately run by a second lab. The difference can be as high as 60 to 80 points.

As I have said since I was a girl, never accept bad news without checking it to make sure it's correct.

If it looks bad, get another test. And if it looks bad the second time, go on the cholesterol-dissolving plan I've just given you, and the third test will thrill you beyond belief.

SUMMARY

Do Eat

- activated charcoal
- apples
- artichokes
- barley
- beans
- beets
- blackberries
- blueberries
- bluefish
- canola oil
- carrots
- chicken
- chili pepper
- cornish hens
- duck
- eggplant
- garlic
- ginger
- goose
- grapefruit
- green tea
- green plaintains
- guggul
- herring
- lemons
- limes
- mackerel
- nuts
- oat bran
- olive oil
- onions
- oranges
- papaya
- pheasant
- pineapple
- reishi mushrooms
- salmon
- sardines
- seafood
- seaweed
- shiitake mushrooms
- sole
- spinach
- strawberries
- sunflower seeds
- tuna
- turkey
- whole wheat
- yogurt

Vitamins And Minerals That Help

- vitamin C   • vitamin E   • niacin

Foods To Be Aware Of!

No more than 30% of your daily calories should come from:

- bacon
- coconut oil
- dairy products:cheese, eggs, whole milk, butter
- fats: saturates, monosaturates, and polysaturates.
- palm oil
- processed meats
- red meat

9

Constipation: The Woman Who Has Discovered Her Second Youth Is Never – But Never – Constipated

*L*et's begin with a workable definition of constipation. This means that you never — but never — will be taken victim again by the crackpot theory that you have to have a bowel movement every day to be healthy. If you have one every two or three days with no strain and feel fine, that is your natural pace and there is absolutely no reason to try and accelerate it. Undue fretting about frequency only creates a problem where none exists.

Be aware that doctors have evolved a clinical definition of constipation: difficult, incomplete, or infrequent evacuation of the bowels (less than three times a week).

But what if you are neither a clinical case nor a hypochondriac obsessed with your bowels, and you just do not feel fine? Do you suffer from the strain, bloating, gas, backaches and headaches associated with constipation? This is unnatural and you don't have to suffer from it a minute longer. Considering

Intestinal blocks do not respond to more fiber, so don't keep packing in more fiber until you have cleaned out the old.

that there are five feet of large intestines and twenty feet of small intestines, you would be much happier if they were kept supple and free from debris.

You have certainly been bombarded with the theory of the high-fiber diet. True, it is very helpful for regularity, cholesterol control and colon cancer prevention. However, intestinal blocks do not respond to more fiber so, if you are having a problem with elimination, don't keep packing in more fiber until you have cleaned out the old.

Here are simple, natural ways to find relief.

Drink and Go Merrily

The easiest way to cure constipation involves no laxatives, no fiber and no money. It simply makes it easy and automatic for your bowels to slide out their waste products. Make sure you drink enough liquids every day to keep the waste products inside you moving along smoothly. Otherwise, the stool becomes too hard for muscular contractions to push it out easily.

These liquids should be primarily water. Just plain, simple, natural, everyday water. And you should drink six to eight glasses a day, every day.

I call it "sipping constipation away." Three easy steps. Any time of the day have a glass of water available where you can simply reach down and sip it. Give yourself water-relaxation breaks every few minutes of that day. Stop what you are doing. Shake out the tightness from your limbs. Stretch. Think mountain spring thoughts, and have another healthy sip. Get back to relaxed regularity in three weeks.

Or, if you wish, you can add herbs or spices once or twice a day to intensify the effect. Here are a few:

- The juice of one lemon in a glass of water on arising and before going to bed is an old remedy for cleaning out the tract.
- Powdered butternut bark stimulates your intestines without gripping or cramping.
- Tea made from dock root — the traditional Chinese treatment for chronic constipation.
- One teaspoon of macerated mustard seeds, taken with a little water, on an empty stomach.
- And the old reliable, chamomile tea, which not only acts as a natural laxative but also gives you a calming effect, especially before you go to sleep.

To Prevent Constipation, Go with the Grain

Nothing beats fiber from whole grains for moving stools. Whole wheat bread and wheat germ are a ready source. In many clinics, nursing homes and hospitals, wheat bran has already replaced laxatives.

A new Swedish study shows that, in elderly patients, constipation was cured by adding fiber-rich crispbreads such as Wasa Fiber. These little crispbreads are made from wheat bran and rye meal, and as little as 2 1/2 to 6 pieces a day did the trick.

If you're allergic to wheat, oats in oatmeal or oat bran muffins also provide the high-fiber content you need. Barley, though less publicized, is equally helpful. Simply add the barley to soups, or use barley flour for biscuits and muffins.

Brewer's yeast is recommended by source after source as well.

In elderly patients, constipation was cured by adding fiber-rich crispbreads such as Wasa Fiber.

To Cure Constipation, Take Your Pulse

Legumes, alias pulse, are another excellent source of fiber. If they are not already staples in your diet, as they should be, please introduce them gradually. Most people believe that beans are the musical fruit, since the more you eat the more you toot. But this is simply not true. Regular bean eaters do not sound off, but if you are unaccustomed to pulse, you may do so at first until your system adjusts.

As with exercise and so many other foods and activities which are great for you, it is a matter of getting used to the new health regime. Start easy. Very, very easy. Have only a spoonful for an entire course at your meal the very first time you try them. Then, gradually, one week at a time, add another spoonful.

Here, as always, building Second Youth is a matter of weeks, not days. But the results are certainly so incredible that this gradualism pays off.

Finally, some types of beans tend to be more audible than others — for example: chickpeas, split peas, navy beans, black beans and lentils. But you must discover this for yourself, as well as which of them you like best.

Vegetables and Fruits That Fight Constipation

Vegetables high in fiber include artichokes, asparagus, broccoli, Brussels sprouts, cabbage, carrots, cauliflower, parsnips, peas, potatoes (with skins), spinach and squash.

These vegetables are cruciferous and can be gas producers, particularly if eaten raw. If you have a spastic colon or sensitive digestive tract, steam or boil them for easier digestion.

Parsley, though primarily a diuretic, has some laxative properties as well. And all seaweeds and sea vegetables help keep you regular.

As for fruit, you do not have to restrict yourself to stewed prunes, unless you like them, or prune juice. Be an apple polisher: an unpeeled apple a day — before breakfast — is a catalyst. Other fruits, dried, stewed, poached or eaten fresh, supply constipation-fighting fiber as well. They include figs, raisins, apricots, bananas, blackberries, blueberries, boysenberries, cranberries, raspberries, strawberries and pears.

> ❖ *PERSONAL NOTE:* I have found that yogurt, my "double-whammy" bedtime snack, works wonders for me in two ways. The natural tryptophan in it makes me sleep like a baby throughout the night. And the acidophilus in it works as a gentle laxative by morning.

Why Food Is Better Than Laxatives

Yes, it's okay to take laxatives in a pinch. For example, constipation can be brought on by travel or unusual stress. But regular, dependent use of laxatives, and relying on commercial, man-made laxatives instead of nature's own constipation healers is a grievous error.

Castor oil, for example, can damage the cells that line your intestinal tract. Other types of laxatives irritate the bowel wall and flush out needed vitamins and minerals such as potassium before they can be absorbed.

Above all, habitual use tends to weaken the intestinal muscles, bringing on lazy bowel syndrome. In other words, after a certain point your bowels function even less than before because the harsh laxatives are doing their job for them.

Please remember, dietary remedies may not work overnight. Your bowels may have to be coaxed along to natural regularity for a while. But, with moder-

Relying on commercial, man-made laxatives instead of nature's own constipation healers is a grievous error.

ate amounts of patience and persistence, foods and liquids are the best ways to regain full and permanent bowel strength.

If you want to take any "laxative" while improving your diet, choose one that is psyllium-based. This is because psyllium is non-addictive and generally safe. There are many brands on the market, but some tend to be too expensive. This can be easily avoided by making your own version. All you need do is grind two parts psyllium seeds to one part flax and one part oat bran.

Enemas Are the Enemy

Many people, more than you would guess, rely on frequent so-called cleansing of the colon with enemas. But these aggravate constipation even more than laxatives. And those enemas containing irritants, such as soapsuds, should absolutely be avoided.

Enemas prescribed as preparations for certain examinations of the colon have a definite purpose and are certainly not advisable as a treatment for constipation.

The same goes for high-colonics, once the rage among health cultists — Mae West allegedly among them, believe it or not.

Other Ways To Loosen Up

Unless circumstances simply don't allow it, do not hold back or resist the urge to move your bowels. The best way to avoid this is to try to make a habit of evacuating at the same time every day. This should be anytime that is absolutely convenient, undisturbed, and comfortable for you.

Also, get in the habit of giving yourself evacuating signals. For example, breakfast coffee and a cigarette have been used for generations. Now we know that the cigarette should be thrown out of that equation, so use only the coffee by itself.

Perhaps the greatest single no-cost constipation elimina-tor is regular physical exercise. It is, of course, good for you in so many ways. It also, almost alone, makes you regular by moving the waste — and the poisons it contains — through your bowels as much as twice as fast.

The basic exercise to cure constipation is just plain, simple walking. Be active — dance in your living room, go swim-ming or bicycling, have sex. Do whatever turns you on to get your bowels moving.

As the body moves, so will the bowels.

The stretches outlined in this book are another good bet, especially if you think tension may be partly responsible for your constipation.

Massage! Just the word alone gives me visions of relaxation and relief from pain. You can massage your intestines very successfully. Here's how:

❖ Lie on your back with your knees up, feet flat on the floor.

Massage your abdomen with your hands, moving in a circular motion.

Start in the center by your belly button and work outward in a circle that gets bigger and bigger.

Go first in a clockwise direction.

Then reverse, and go in a counter-clockwise direc-tion.

If you feel a lump or painful knot, let your fingers rest firmly on it until it softens. It is probably a gas pocket that can be moved along by your gentle knead-ing.

Belly dancing does wonders, if that is your bent. And yoga abdominal movements foster intestinal function. Here is the best one:

❖ Sit cross-legged. Concentrate on your abdominal muscles. Rotate them, without using your hands, in a circular movement from right to left. Then reverse the roll, and move them from left to right.

Don't worry too much if you don't get much movement at first. The more you do it, the better you'll be at it.

Another wonderful yoga exercise that massages your abdomen from inside:

❖ Sit or stand with your knees slightly bent.
Place your hands on your knees or mid-thighs.
Blow all your air out, then suck your belly in. You will feel all your abdominal muscles engaging in this effort. Using your muscles, push your abdomen out and pull it back in, without taking a breath. See how many out-and-in movements you can do before you feel the need to take a breath. You may be able to do only six or seven pulses, but your muscle control will improve with practice.

This exercise will also help to flatten your tummy and stimulate your vital organs.

According to Alison Crane, R.N., president of the American Association for Therapeutic Humor, a good belly laugh helps. In addition to immediately relieving stress, it "massages" the intestines. So while you may protest that constipation is no laughing matter, anything that gets you rolling in the aisles may be all for the best.

When To See A Doctor

You should see your doctor at once if constipation has never been a problem before and it suddenly and stubbornly sets in. You need to have it ruled out, or spotted early, as a symptom of an underlying disease.

Moreover, if you are taking drugs to treat depression, hypertension, Parkinson's disease or heart disorders, be aware that some of them trigger constipation. If this cause and effect relationship occurs in your life as the result of a new prescription, for example, speak to your doctor about a change of medication. This may be all you need to eliminate the unwanted side effect.

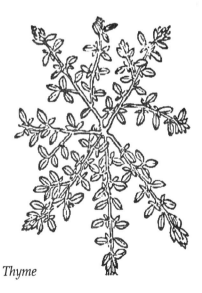

Thyme

SUMMARY

Remedies for Constipation
Liquids (Water, Juices). Mix With:

- chamomile tea
- dock root tea
- lemon
- macerated mustard seeds
- powdered butternut bark

Grains

- barley
- bran
- brewer's yeast
- oats
- rye
- whole wheat

Legumes

- beans
- chickpeas
- lentils
- split peas

Fruits

- apples
- apricots
- bananas
- blackberries
- blueberries
- boysenberries
- cranberries
- figs
- pears
- prunes
- raisins
- raspberries
- strawberries

Vegetables

- artichokes
- asparagus
- broccoli
- brussels sprouts
- cabbage
- carrots
- cauliflower
- celery
- parsley
- parsnips
- peas
- potatoes
- seaweed
- spinach
- squash

Other Remedies

- active sports
- exercise
- hobbies
- laughter!
- massage
- psyllium
- yoga
- yogurt

10

Diabetes: Natural Healers that Treat and Prevent Diabetes

*I*f you have diabetes, this chapter will help you live better with it and ward off some of its most disastrous consequences.

If you do not now have diabetes (to your knowledge – I'll explain in a moment), then this chapter will help you prevent contracting it in the middle stage of your life.

You see, it is estimated that some 14 million Americans suffer from diabetes. This makes it the fourth leading cause of death by disease in the United States. But the frightening fact is that almost *half* may not even know they have it. They do not realize that it can start in middle age, and not just when they are young.

Left unrecognized and untreated, diabetes makes you particularly prone to heart disease and stroke, blindness, kidney failure and gangrene. With it, whether you know you have it or not, simple infections can pose unexpected risks.

Yet you need not suffer from any one of these dire consequences! In the case of adult-onset diabetes — the diabetes that strikes only when you have reached full maturity — you may not even need medication. Often you can control the disease through food alone. Let me explain.

If you develop diabetes when you are a child, then your pancreas fails to produce insulin, the essential hormone for glucose (sugar) absorption. But if you develop diabetes when you are an adult, your body still produces the needed insulin, but becomes unable to fully use it without help. And you have that help at your fingertips!

In the face of these facts, what do you do right now? It's simple. First, make sure that you have a yearly visit with your doctor, and that he tests your blood sugar to see if you have hidden diabetes.

If you don't, then go on to the next chapter. But if you do, fight this adult-onset diabetes with the following delicious foods.

Strict Diets for Diabetes Are Out

Over the years, diet prescriptions for diabetics have swerved between high and low consumption of calories, carbohydrates, protein or fat. Nowadays, however, it is recognized that these stern restrictive plans just do not work, and also that no one diet can be correct for all people because their conditions vary.

For example, until recently, sugar and other simple carbohydrates were an absolute no-no. The thinking was that since high-glucose levels in the blood are characteristic of diabetes, you must not eat sugars. However, current guidelines, though far from an invitation to overindulge, permit up to five percent of calories to come from simple carbohydrates.

There is, however, a trick to eating these simple carbohydrates. Your body absorbs them far more easily when they are part of a meal that contains fruit, vegetables, meat, fowl or fish. In other words, don't just take a glass of orange juice, a sugary soft drink or candy by itself, with nothing else along-side it. This will produce an unwanted surge in your blood glucose.

Instead have, for example, an occasional ice cream for dessert. This will produce far less of a rise because the food you have eaten just before will buffer it in your system.

Overweight Is Out
But Fat Can Still Be Part of Your Diet

Once upon a time, high-fat diets were recommended because fats neutralized blood sugar. Not anymore! While fats may have that effect, if you eat a lot of them, especially saturated fats, we now know that you are contributing to high blood cholesterol, arteriosclerosis and heart disease — all of which you, as a diabetic, are extremely vulnerable to.

In addition, because fats contain more calories per gram than carbohydrates and protein, they make weight control more difficult. And, by now everyone knows that obesity aggravates adult-onset dia-betes.

So what do you do? You certainly do not have to swear off all butter, cream and mayonnaise, much less monosatu-rated olive oil. However, your *total* fat intake should not exceed 30 percent of your calories daily. This, as you now know, is the maximum doctors recom-mend for everyone. But for you, it is a matter of life and death.

Just to be on the safe, safe side, I would recommend that you keep it closer to 20 percent to 25 percent for the rest of your life. It's certainly not hard when you consider all the delicious foods you can eat instead.

Your *total* fat intake should not exceed 30 % of your calories daily. For the diabetic, it's a matter of life and death.

> Fiber slows digestion and absorbs water. A fiber-rich, high complex-carbohydrate diet protects the heart health of diabetics.

Fiber Offsets Diabetes

The National Diabetes Associations of the United States, Canada and Great Britain have all endorsed a high fiber diet. Why? Because, by slowing the digestion of simple carbohydrates, fiber may decrease the rise in blood sugar levels after meals. Also, because it absorbs water, fiber gives a sense of fullness, so you are less tempted to overeat and get fat.

Now listen to this! According to James W. Anderson, M.D., professor at the University of Kentucky School of Medicine, a fiber-rich, high complex-carbohydrate diet not only protects the heart health of diabetics, *it is the most important discovery since insulin injections.*

Think of it! Once again, foods, not drugs, are the most important discovery since insulin!

But remember, when you start a fiber diet, start it gently and slowly. Very little at first, then a little more, then even a little more until you work your way up to full-size daily portions.

Gradual. Gradual. Gradual. This way you get the benefits you want, without the gas and bloating you certainly don't want. Load up, but don't overload.

Also, if you're going to try commercial brand products — muffins, for example — read every word on the label. Many of them are loaded with harmful additives. Watch for the danger words I've given you above. Get only a product that swears on its label it is pure bran with nothing disastrous added.

Another luscious way to get your daily fiber is to put beans, potatoes, pasta and whole grains on your plate. Beans, dried peas and lentils are wonderful insulin regulators. Diabetes specialists all over the world now acknowledge a scientific basis for their therapeutic use. They also tend to delay the emptying out of your stomach, causing a slower rise in your blood sugar. And, if you eat them daily, they are helpful in reducing the amount of medication needed in juvenile diabetes, and can virtually eliminate the need for injections in adult-onset diabetes.

Bulgur, which is wheat that has been parboiled, dried and cracked, is also thought to be especially helpful.

Raw Foods Relieve Diabetes

Raw foods, including seeds and nuts, may decrease or eliminate the need for insulin, according to Dr. John M. Douglass, of the Southern California Permanente Medical Group and Kaiser Foundation in Los Angeles.

Among many examples are almonds, apples, blackberries, melons, peanuts, plums, prunes and raisins. In a test of 50 foods, peanuts ranked best on the glycemic index scale, which is a measurement of how fast blood sugar rises after eating. Apples were a close second.

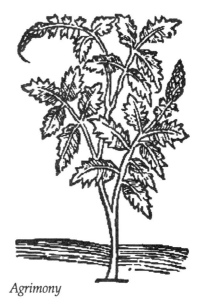

Agrimony

Is This the Missing Mineral that Keeps Your Body From Absorbing Its Precious Insulin?

Many studies, including those done by Dr. Walter Merz, chief of the United States Department of Agriculture's vitamin and mineral research division, have indicated that a shortage of the trace mineral chromium occurs in adult-onset diabetes.

The mounting evidence suggests that chromium helps restore your body's sensitivity to insulin, thus enabling a better metabolism of glucose.

While only small quantities of chromium are needed, they make a difference — perhaps a huge difference — in controlling the disease.

Foods, herbs and spices that contain chromium include:

- black pepper
- blackstrap molasses
- brewer's yeast
- brown rice
- chicken
- cloves
- corn oil
- honey
- parsley
- seaweed
- thyme
- whole wheat

Chromium food supplements based in yeast are also available, with a potency of 200 micrograms per tablet. One a day has been found to be perfectly effective.

The Vitamin That Speeds Up Healing In Your Entire Body

As a diabetic, you are not only vulnerable to infections, but you heal slowly if you have a wound. Vitamin A speeds both these healing processes if it is taken at above normal nutritional requirements.

In immunity especially, some of the very best specialists now believe it should be administered in high dosages to all diabetics. (I'll show you how to get it below.)

Also, to quote Sheldon Saul Hendler, M.D., Ph.D.:

"Just as supplemental vitamin A improves immune responses of traumatized animals and surgical patients, it will be especially useful in preventing wound infection and promoting wound healing in surgical diabetic patients."

To get higher dosages of vitamin A, however, you should do it the safest way. High dosages of vitamin A can be toxic, and therefore you do not want to take them directly. However, what you can do with perfect safety and effectiveness is include plenty of beta-carotene in your diet.

Beta-carotene is a precursor of vitamin A. The body converts as much of it as it needs into vitamin A. Therefore it is non-toxic. And it is also readily available at your greengrocer.

The fruits and vegetables richest in beta-carotene are all yellow and orange. Go for apricots, cantaloupe, carrots, mangoes, papaya, sweet potatoes, pumpkin and butternut squash. But you need not be monochromatic: green leafy vegetables such as collard and dandelion greens, kale, spinach and watercress also provide good sources of beta-carotene.

In addition, I'd really recommend a beta-carotene supplement. You should buy one that has the equivalent of 10,000 units of vitamin A and take one pill every day. You can find it in any health food store.

Any vascular disease diabetics contract is more threatening. Therefore, you need more than average doses of vitamin C.

The Role of Vitamin C

If you're a diabetic, any vascular disease you may contract becomes accelerated, speeded-up, more threatening. Therefore, Dr. George V. Mann of Vanderbilt University is convinced that you need more than average doses of vitamin C. In his opinion, the tiny wounds that so often hinder circulation in your blood vessels reflect a deficiency of vitamin C, much like scurvy in people who do not have diabetes.

Food sources are cantaloupe, citrus fruits, kiwi, papaya, peppers (red bell as well as chili), strawberries and many green vegetables.

In addition, I recommend that you take 500 mg of vitamin C in pill form every day for the first two or three weeks. Then, if you are comfortable with that, double it to 1,000 mg a day from then on.

Nutrients That Save Diabetics' Eyes

Studies in England and Japan show that too little magnesium could be a cause of the pinpoint hemorrhages in the back of the retina which afflict the majority of people who have been diabetic for 20 years or more. As a precautionary measure, eat foods rich in magnesium — whole grains, nuts and dark green leafy vegetables.

Vitamin E and selenium are also helpful. Israeli research shows that, by inhibiting platelet clumping and improving circulation, vitamin E may also offset the damage of these pinpoint hemorrhages. I take a supplement of Vitamin E with selenium every day.

Furthermore, animal studies conducted by John Trevithick, professor of biochemistry at the University of Western Ontario, indicate that vitamin E can almost totally prevent cataracts in diabetic rats.

Finally, bioflavonoid supplements have been found to forestall the painful build-up of fluids in diabetic eyes. Scientists at the National Eye Institute in Bethesda, Maryland, have discovered that one of them, quercitrin, has held off cataracts in diabetic laboratory animals.

Take 400 mg of vitamin E a day, one selenium tablet and a vitamin B-complex supplement per day.

Vitamins That Keep You on Your Toes

Vitamin B^1 (thiamine) and vitamin E supplements have been proposed for the foot problems that plague many older diabetics. Stanley Mirsky, M.D., prescribes thiamine for patients kept awake at night by pain in their feet. He and Harvey Walker, M.D., Ph.D. in Clayton, Missouri also prescribe vitamin E — and Dr. Walker adds lecithin — to maintain good circulation in the feet.

Naturalists' Ways To Allay Diabetes

To treat diabetes, Orientals have long used dong quai and ginseng. For adult-onset diabetes, doctors in Colonia La Raza have found that a common Mexican food, broiled cactus stem, lowers blood glucose levels. These cactus stems also grow in the southwestern United States. In your health food store they may be called opuntia streptacantha.

Here are more proven folk remedies you may also want to try: dandelions for stabilizing blood sugar swings; garlic for detoxifying the body and ridding it of the yeast infections to which diabetics are prone (because they thrive in a high-sugar environment); or tea made from blueberry or huckleberry leaves.

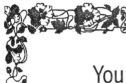

You must exercise. Exercise is one of the best tonics in the world — not only specifically for diabetes, but for your overall health and Second Youth.

Keep Moving, But Watch Your Step

By itself alone, regular exercise improves your ability to handle glucose. In addition, it is an indispensable part of any sensible weight reduction program and especially in the case of adult-onset diabetes, where shedding excess pounds has been proved over and over again to lower blood sugar levels, exercise simply has to be part of your life.

The exercise need not be strenuous. In fact, it probably should never be, because overdoing it can cause an insulin reaction. Much depends, of course, on your age and the overall shape you are in. Check with your doctor or physiotherapist to see if the regime of your choice is okay for you.

Stay away from jarring exercises such as jogging, jumping rope or weightlifting. In addition, if you are older and have a circulatory problem, you should avoid any sport or other activity that is hard on your feet, and after each session keep a close watch on them for bruises, blisters, scratches and cuts.

What this means, quite simply, is get the right exercising footwear. This is a must. You must exercise. Exercise is one of the best tonics in the world for you — not only specifically for diabetes, but for your overall health and Second Youth. The right footwear makes all this possible without risk of any downside or injury.

Symptoms of Adult-Onset Diabetes

- excessive thirstiness
- excessive hunger
- overweight
- dehydration
- blurred vision
- dizziness
- nausea and vomiting
- labored breathing

Many of these symptoms, of course, could indicate causes other than adult-onset diabetes. But if you have two or more, why not check in with your doctor?

SUMMARY

Foods To Eat

Fiber-Rich Foods

- almonds
- apples
- beans
- blackberries
- bulgur
- dried peas
- lentils
- melons
- pasta
- peanuts
- plums
- potatoes
- prunes
- raisins
- whole grains

Beta Carotene/Vitamin A Foods

- apricots
- butternut squash
- cantaloupe
- carrots
- collard greens
- dandelion greens
- kale
- mangoes
- papaya
- pumpkin
- spinach
- sweet potatoes
- watercress

Vitamin C Foods

- cantaloupe
- citrus fruits
- green vegetables
- kiwi
- papaya
- peppers
- strawberries

Chromium-Rich Foods

- black pepper
- blackstrap molasses
- brewer's yeast
- brown rice
- cloves
- chicken
- corn oil
- honey
- parsley
- seaweed
- thyme
- whole wheat

Magnesium-Rich Foods

- bioflavonoid supplements – also found in the white fiber of citrus fruits
- dark green leafy vegetables
- nuts
- selenium with vitamin E supplements
- vitamin B^1/thiamine supplements
- whole grains

Naturalists' Remedies

- broiled cactus stems (also known as opuntia streptacantha)
- dong quai
- ginseng
- dandelions
- garlic
- blueberry leaf tea
- huckleberry leaf tea

Other Remedies

- Exercise with your doctor's approval
- Have no more than 20-25% of your daily calories in fat
- Have no more than 5% of your daily calories in simple carbohydrates (taken only with a full meal)

11

Diarrhea: How To Conquer Diarrhea as Quickly and Painlessly as Possible

Surely, at one time or another you have had this malady. Because it is so common, especially among travelers, a rich array of non-medical names for it exists: the runs, the trots, Lucy Bowel, the Cairo curse, Delhi belly, Hong Kong dog, Montezuma's revenge, and turista.

Diarrhea can be triggered by food poisoning, rotaviruses, or just eating or drinking something that "disagrees" with you. Other less frequent causes are medications, such as antibiotics or antacids containing magnesium, excess vitamin C, or overuse of foods and beverages that contain the artificial sweetener sorbitol. In some people, as we all know, stress or anxiety loosens the bowels, just as in others, it provokes headaches.

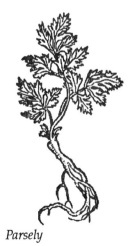

Parsely

Most attacks are short-lived. They are your body's way of getting rid of something nasty. The best cure is to let them run their course and peter out.

The Very Best Way To Deal With Diarrhea

Most diarrhea attacks are short-lived, and the best cure is simply to let them run their course and peter out. According to Lynn V. McFarland, a research associate with the Department of Medicinal Chemistry at the University of Washington, they are your body's way of getting rid of something nasty.

That is all well and good if you are at leisure — though, even then, you do not want to be chained to the toilet. What if you have pressing engagements or your holiday trip will be ruined, and you simply cannot go with the flow?

Non-Prescription Healers

Many doctors recommend *Immodium*, an over-the-counter drug that comes in both capsule and liquid form. Alternatives for mild diarrhea include *Kaopectate* and *Pepto-Bismol*. I would, therefore, store one of these in your medicine cabinet, and take it along when traveling. Activated charcoal tablets, sold in most pharmacies as well as health food stores, are also believed to curb bacterial growth. The usual dose for diarrhea is two to three tablets every eight hours.

Liquids Are Vital

If diarrhea starts, the most essential thing is to keep your fluid intake high in order to counteract dehydration (no, an increase in fluids will *not* make you go more). Liquids that also contain salt and sugar to replace lost glucose and minerals are best and honey may be better than sugar. Recommended formulas include the following:

1. Add a teaspoon of sugar or honey and a pinch of salt to one quart of bottled mineral water or boiled tap water (drink only bottled or boiled water, of course). Use a mineral water that is flat rather than bubbly, because the gas in carbonated beverages can be irritating. Drink the water over the course of the day.

2. Mix one-half teaspoon of salt, one-half teaspoon of baking soda and four teaspoons of sugar or honey in a quart of safe water. Drink over the course of the day.

3. Mix one-half teaspoon of honey and a pinch of salt in eight ounces of fruit juice. Repeat several times a day.

4. This is the World Health Organization's remedy for travelers: add a pinch of salt and one-half teaspoon of honey to an eight-ounce glass of orange juice. Add one-quarter teaspoon of baking soda to another eight-ounce glass filled with distilled water. Alternate drinking from each glass. Be sure to squeeze the juice yourself, or watch it being squeezed from the whole fruit.

5. Add a pinch each of cayenne pepper and cinnamon to two cups of boiling water. Simmer for 20 minutes. Allow to cool and take two tablespoons every hour.

6. Sip clear liquids such as broths and sweetened boiled tea.

Bananas
not
only
contain
pectin,
which
can
tighten
loose
bowels,
but
they
restore
needed
minerals
often
lost
in
diarrhea,
such
as
magnesium
and
potassium.

Curative Foods

The Zen approach is to eat nothing in order to re-establish healthy bowels by resting your digestive system. While this may be too severe for you, food intake should be kept strictly on the bland side at first. When diarrhea strikes, you are liable to feel skittish about eating anyway. Or, you may only want such easy-to-swallow, soothing foods as jellied consommé or soft-boiled eggs.

A classic Italian grandmother's remedy is rice, served with some of the water it was boiled in.

Yogurt and/or tablets containing lactobacillus acidophilus are of great help, particularly if the diarrhea is caused by antibiotics such as penicillin, or infectious agents. Yogurt's ability to recolonize friendly bacteria in your intestinal tract is widely known.

Bananas not only contain pectin, which can tighten loose bowels, but they restore needed minerals often lost in diarrhea, such as magnesium and potassium.

To benefit from both, chop two bananas in a pint of plain yogurt, add one tablespoon of fiber, mix and enjoy.

Another food you may consider is blueberries, a common Swedish folk remedy for diarrhea. Eat them plain or try mixing them with yogurt instead of bananas.

Foods containing protease inhibitors — soybeans, in particular — were found by researchers at the Johns Hopkins University School of Medicine to subdue rotaviruses that cause diarrhea.

Beware of Coffee and Milk

Lactose intolerance, which can begin at any age, is thought to be a leading cause of diarrhea in this country. Just because you have always drunk milk with no ill effects does not mean that you will always tolerate it. Milk drinkers who suddenly start having spates of diarrhea are advised to abstain from milk products for a week or two, and see if it makes a difference.

Coffee can also activate or aggravate chronic diarrhea, due perhaps to its caffeine content. Cutting back or completely eliminating its consumption on an experimental basis is certainly worth a try.

Do Not Let a Trip Trip You Up

When you travel to countries where the food, drink, sanitary standards and climate are different from those at home, you are particularly susceptible to the kind of diarrhea caused by Escheria coli bacteria. That does not mean that you should not try local dishes. They are one of the pleasures of traveling. It all depends on the particular country, and what and how you eat there.

Here are the basic rules. They are simple, but stick strictly to them.

1. Watch out for the water. Unless you are sure it is safe, do not drink water from a tap, well or stream without sterilizing it. How do you make it safe? Iodine tablets or crystals will kill most microbes, but you may not have any handy. Boiling tap water for 15 minutes — no less — usually will disinfect it enough. If you have any deep fears, try 20 minutes.

In countries far enough above the tropics, it is okay to use unboiled water to brush your teeth, as long as you do not swallow it. However, I use only bottled water to brush mine, because the trip is much too precious to me to risk it, even with this simple action.

Avoid all ice in beverages, alcoholic or not. If the water used to make the ice is contaminated, as that ice melts it will release bacteria into your drink. Do not count on the alcohol killing the germs. It simply cannot in that temperature.

2. Avoid raw foods such as salad greens. Simply avoid them. Say "*No*" to them in any form. Vegetables and fruits that can be peeled just before you eat them are okay, but see them being peeled with your own eyes and be sure they have been washed in the iodine solution before peeling to prevent the transfer of bacteria to the peeled food.

3. Avoid raw shellfish almost anywhere. By now, due to pollution, that includes most places in the United States and Europe, not just in the Third World. What a loss, what a shame! But you must face this reality.

❖ PERSONAL NOTE: I have done a lot of traveling in areas that have unsafe sanitary conditions as described above. However, my experience has been that the modern hotels catering to tourists are very sanitary in their preparation of food. Don't hesitate to ask, if you have any doubts.

When To Call a Doctor

Usually, you will find that the diarrhea stops by itself, without your consulting a doctor. However, you must call the doctor if:

- the diarrhea does not stop within two or three days
- it is accompanied by fever and severe abdominal cramps
- it produces yellowing of the skin and whites of the eyes
- it causes blood, pus, or mucus in your stools
- it results in weakness

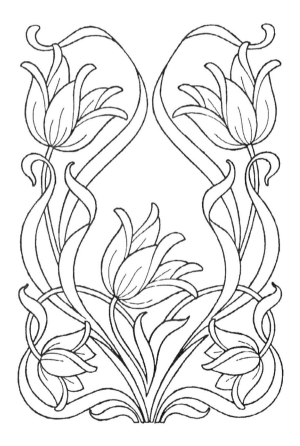

Summary

Over-The-Counter Help

- activated charcoal tablets
- Immodium
- Kaopectate
- Pepto-Bismol

Nature's Helpers

- bananas
- blueberries
- bottled water or boiled water
- cayenne pepper and cinnamon in water
- freshly squeezed orange juice
- jellied consomme
- plenty of fluids that contain salt and sugar or honey
- rice
- soft-boiled eggs
- soybeans
- tea with sugar
- yogurt

Avoid

- caffeine in coffee and chocolate drinks
- ice in drinks when traveling
- milk products if you have a lactose intolerance
- raw shellfish
- raw vegetables and salads when traveling
- unboiled water when traveling in other countries

12

Headaches: Second Youth Freedom From Headaches

$\mathcal{A}$ ccording to the National Headache Foundation, three out of four Americans had a headache during the past year. To my way of thinking, that's far too many.

Usually, of course, a minor headache is no big deal. You take an aspirin, have a cup of coffee, put an ice pack on your forehead, meditate or go for a walk, and the pain usually goes away.

But, as you know, there are headaches, and there are *headaches!* What is an occasional passing annoyance for most people, is torture for far too many others. Chronic tension, cluster or migraine headaches are said to account for 40 to 80 million doctor visits every year. They cost our society about 157 million workdays every year.

> ❖ PERSONAL NOTE: This comes as no surprise to me. Migraines first attacked me as a child, and plagued my life relentlessly. It is only in recent years that I learned how to deal with them without medication.

The First Steps Toward Self-Help
For Chronic Headaches

Though chronic headaches vary in type, there are measures you can take that seem to help any kind instantly. They are these:

Keep a headache diary. This will tell you the triggers of your headaches. It's very simple. Simply put down each day the time, place, etc. of each attack. What were you doing? In what position? Who were you with? What medications are you taking?

The last question is especially important. For example, if you take drugs for headache relief too often, they can wind up causing those headaches rather than erasing them. Also, oral contraceptives or hormone replacement therapy, nasal sprays, decongestants, appetite suppressants and certain diuretics could be the triggers you are looking for.

Do your headaches happen mostly at work, or during the weekdays? Do they coincide with a change in barometric pressure or wind conditions? Are they worse when you lie down . . . sit down . . . bend over? Do you wake up with them? Do you experience constipation at the same time? Are you bloated?

Do you have the proper indoor lighting? The proper indoor ventilation? Do you chew gum? This may seem like a dumb question, but constant chewing can overwork jaw muscles, leading to what is called reflex headaches.

What did you have to eat or drink that day, and the day before? This is especially important. Why? Because foods and food additives play a major role in many headaches, especially migraines.

Therefore, in your headache diary jot down every morsel of food or drink that you consumed that day. Be sure to include the condiments, salt and spices. Try this for at least two or three weeks. Then you will automatically see what led up to each of your headaches.

You are looking for a pattern. For similar causes. For the triggers that set off your headaches, time and time again. In 9 out of 10 cases, this diary will show you in those two or three weeks where your headaches are coming from, and therefore how they can be avoided.

Once you have established a trigger, or several triggers, you can then go about avoiding them. If they are a particular food or foods, for example, you can simply cut them out of your diet.

However, if they are an emotional reaction, you may not be able to avoid such triggers as traffic jams, your boss, or recurrent family problems. But you can know the physical toll these problems take on you. And you can try to lower the emotional level in such situations, or institute a series of brief relaxation exercises in order to interrupt the emotional problem-headache cycle.

Of course, more than one trigger may be involved. See if you can eliminate one, and ameliorate the other. What you are really trying to do is this: You want to see what causes the headaches . . . what triggers them off . . . so you can then take action against them.

Ways To Feed a Headache So It Goes Away

There has been extremely thrilling news about migraines in scientific research over the past few years. Here is what they found:

There is good evidence that omega-3 fish oil capsules, calcium and magnesium supplements are of vast benefit to headache sufferers of all types.

Before a migraine strikes, there is what is called a pre-migraine phase. You probably know it as the feeling, or warning, of an approaching attack. There may be squiggly lights floating in your peripheral vision which are known as the "aura." Or a blackout in the center of your vision. You may feel pressure in your head, as though it was filled with too much fluid.

Doctors have now found that this pressure comes from increased platelet aggregation — in other words, from blood thickening in your brain.

Let's look at a recent study in the *Journal of the American Medical Association*. It was written by Donald J. Dalessio, M.D., of the Scripps Clinic and Research Foundation in La Jolla, California. And his results strongly suggest that this thickening of the blood, which he calls a tendency toward clotting, may explain why migraine patients have a slightly higher incidence of stroke.

Clearly, therefore, any substance that interferes with platelet aggregation could be protective against both migraines and strokes.

One that certainly does this is vitamin E. Therefore, try 400 mg of vitamin E each day.

Other research has linked low blood sugar to migraines. Two recent reports were published in the *New England Journal of Medicine* and *Headache Magazine*. They suggest that you start a high-protein, sugar-free regime. But, in this case, try to do it in five or six small meals, rather than the standard three meals a day.

In other words, don't let your blood sugar get so low that it explodes your cranium.

There is good evidence that omega-3 fish oil capsules, calcium and magnesium supplements are of vast benefit to headache sufferers of all types. Also, a diet rich in leafy green vegetables to ensure enough intake of iron.

In his books, Carlson Wade, enzyme catalyst maven, recommended drinking a glass of fresh cabbage, celery, lettuce or any green vegetable juice immediately upon the onset of a sudden headache.

For recurring headaches, he also prescribed at least one raw food meal on alternate days. And he emphasized citrus fruits or their juices for sinus headaches in particular.

Now let's look at a proven, effective homeopathic remedy. It is seaweed, and it is often used to treat headaches in homeopathic medicine. Powdered or fresh ginger has been said to stop a migraine in its tracks when taken at the onset of the aura, and then at 4-hour intervals the same day. I have a little ginger in every day's diet as a headache preventive.

A very old folk remedy for migraine is feverfew, also known as bachelor's button. Now, not surprisingly, the Queen's Medical Centre, in Nottingham, England, confirms its effectiveness. It can be taken in tablet form, available in your health food store.

Powdered or fresh ginger has been said to stop a migraine in its tracks when taken at the onset of the aura, and then at 4-hour intervals the same day.

And there are the herbal tisanes and infusions, such as peppermint, rosemary, catnip and sage. The best way to take them is to sip them quietly, and then lie down in as complete relaxation as possible for 20 minutes.

I know you can't always do this, but it works perfectly for me to separate a hard day from a marvelous night.

Why Coffee Can Be Both Good and Bad For Headaches

I swear by coffee to clear my head in the morning. I rarely drink it after that, but one or two cups for breakfast make a big difference. This is particularly true on muggy, overcast or rainy days, another prime time for migraine in my life. When the barometer is low, I wake up feeling like my head is full of water and my brain may be in danger of drowning. Coffee has diuretic properties and therefore clears that up, and peps me up as well.

At the ashram near New York where I used to retreat, I had sickening, horrible migraines the first two or three days I was there, and could not figure out why. An ashram is an oasis of peace and serenity, but for those first two days it was exactly the opposite for me.

Finally, it dawned on me that I was going through caffeine withdrawal. Neither coffee nor tea were served, only herbal teas.

Therefore, this particular aspect of the yoga regime did not fit my own physiology. I corrected it immediately, and my philosophy now is very simple. If a few cups of coffee help me ward off migraine, I see every reason to have them, and none whatsoever to abstain.

On the one hand, caffeine constricts blood vessels, thus making it invaluable in the treatment of migraines, but on the other hand, too much caffeine can *cause* headaches instead of dissipating them. For example, a broker friend of mine attributed his constant jitters and tension headaches, which he had not had before, to the lay-offs and retrenchments on Wall Street after the excesses of the 80's. His new, smaller office was closer to the coffee machine than the water cooler. His jitters and headaches stopped when he realized that he was sipping coffee all day as if it were bottled spring water and stopped the practice.

Here is a list of foods you must test to see if they are your headache triggers

The most common triggers for headaches, especially migraines, are foods that contain tyramine. These include:

- avocados
- bananas
- dairy products like aged cheese
- figs
- ice cream
- sour cream

As you know only too well, ice cream can set off a headache because its cold activates the nerves in the roof of your mouth.

Others triggers are:

- chocolate
- citrus fruits
- nuts
- navy beans
- eggplant
- pickled herring
- soy sauce
- beef and chicken livers
- cured meats
- wheat
- red wine

I know this is a long list, but each week eliminate one at a time from your diet and see if you feel better at the very end of the week.

It is no excuse for you to say that you have never been sensitive to these foods before. Sensitivity can grow as you grow older. As you hit your 40's and 50's for example, foods that never, never bothered you before may suddenly explode a blinding headache.

This is one of the prices we pay for surviving so long. But that "survival" can be beautiful, if only we can go along with the changes, rather than fight or ignore them, and eliminate those that now give us trouble.

Part of the problem with cured meats such as hot dogs, bacon, ham, salami and sausage may be the nitrates and nitrites used to preserve them. These foods are also salty, and that's not very good for your headache either.

Dr. J.B. Brainard, who suffered for years from migraines, finally realized that they mostly occurred after he ate very salty foods. He immediately switched to a low-sodium diet and was vastly relieved. So much so, in fact, that he recommended the same switch to many of his surgery patients who also had a history of migraines and who also immediately obtained the same great relief.

Other well-known triggers are the flavor-enhancer monosodium glutamate (MSG) and sulfites.

Again, do not try to banish all of these substances in one fell swoop. That would be ridiculous. Instead, eliminate them one by one over a period of a week to two weeks, and see if you can feel the difference in a reduction of the number and intensity of your headaches.

You may already have learned to solve some of the problems, because the cause-effect link for you is clear. I know, for instance, that I was not able to drink red wine — not at all — without paying for it the next day in severe headache pain. But somehow the chemical change in my body during the last two years has now rid me of that trigger, and today I can drink a maximum of two glasses of red wine without the backlash of another headache. You may also be able to drink it with impunity.

Citrus fruits, as another example, often are helpful rather than harmful. But you must test them individually, as with all these other foods.

Trial and experiment is the key. Only then can you tell what to avoid.

Meanwhile, do not skip meals. Do not have simply a danish and coffee for breakfast. Do not put off lunch because of work pressure. Do not have an inadequate dinner because you do not like to eat alone. All of these common habits are horrors for your head because hunger is a notorious trigger for headaches. Give yourself time to be well.

Mind Over Matter for Migraines

Migraines can come at any time and they certainly may be hereditary. All of my family and relatives suffer from them. And unfortunately, they are more common in women than men.

Lewis Carroll, who suffered from severe migraines, is said to have drawn part of his inspiration for *Alice in Wonderland* from the visual distortions that signaled his attacks. Few of us have such powers of imagination, but all of us can use our minds to vanquish pain.

When I was about to get a migraine, my center of vision went black. I could have been looking straight at you and not seen you. Then all around the black hole, squiggles like little worms started crawling. I shall never forget the horror of those recurrent experiences.

Other people have other reactions — they might sense lights flashing in their heads or their hands might turn icy cold.

And these signals are no less clear in a darkened room. In fact, if you are like I was, the onset of a migraine can wake you up from a sound sleep. I attributed this to the stress I had built up during the day, that was being replayed in my dreams.

When I awakened, for example, my neck was almost always in a tense position.

What I learned to do — and this was the secret that probably freed me from these horrors — was to immediately change position. Coax my body into more or less complete relaxation and then start to picture in my mind that all my muscles were relaxed, and that the blood was flowing ever so smoothly through the vessels in my head where I felt the pain.

Eventually, after trying this over and over again, the attacks of migraine would dissipate and I would almost immediately go back to sleep.

By the way, if you tend to get migraines in bed as I did, never sleep turtle fashion, pulling the covers over your head, because that reduces the flow of oxygen to your brain.

What should you do when a migraine strikes at work, or in busy, public places? Use the same visualization and relaxation technique at once. Of course this isn't easy to do, but you can put it to work without the people around you having any idea you are doing so.

If you are sitting, continue sitting where you are, but stop everything you are doing. Concentrate, not on your head, but on your hands. At first, they will feel cold. This is an excellent sign, because if you can warm them up, you will have to draw the blood away from your throbbing head. Biofeedback therapy works on this premise.

If possible, close your eyes. Concentrate all your awareness on those poor cold hands of yours. Put yourself, in your imagination, on the most beautiful beach you have ever seen. Feel the hot sun beating down on those hands as they lie by your sides on that beautiful beach.

Feel the warmth begin to sink into every molecule of your hands. Feel the sun warm your hands so much that you instinctively begin to look for another coating of suntan oil.

Feel your hands tingle. They are becoming hotter and hotter every single minute.

Now they are becoming so hot that you almost want to pick them up and blow on them. They are pulsating with warmth. You could fry an egg on them.

Feel . . . feel . . . feel the heat. Think about nothing but those hot little hands. Forget your head and the pain that was in it a moment before. The more you focus on your hands, the less pain there will be left in your head. The particles of pain are picked up by the blood leaving your head, then floated into your hands and on into the room surrounding you.

This imaging can be done on a crowded street, the subway, a bus, a taxi, or anywhere else you may find yourself when a migraine is starting to strike. After a week or two of practice, you can do it with your eyes open just as well as with them closed. You can even drive a car with full awareness of the road, and still feel your hands drawing the pain out of your head.

However, if you do feel a migraine coming, it is best, of course, to get off the road if you are driving and stay still until the pain subsides.

If you are home, it is a very good idea to put an ice pack on your head and another at the base of your skull. The same principle of staying still also applies here.

Then, there are always the greatest weapons you ever had against headache pain of any kind — your legs. Use them when the pain begins to mount up. Walk. Or walk rapidly. Or jog. This reduces your headache pain by a very simple remedy: it increases the flow of the brain chemical endorphin which destroys the pain particles.

> The greatest weapons against headache pain of any kind – your legs. Use them when the pain begins to mount up.

Remedies for Chronic Tension Headaches

Chronic tension causes chronic pain. One of the ways that pain can show itself is through headaches.

Chronic tension headaches are a bad habit which you have allowed to seize control of your body. Of course the tension is there. Of course you have to live through it. But everything depends on the way you live through it.

When you are under a siege of tension — and which of us is not under a terrible siege of tension every single week — you must say this to yourself.

> "I have been through situations like this before. Yes, they are bad. But I have survived them. And I will survive this.
>
> "And I will survive them better if I do not let their tension rot my body and rot my brain. No one here can hurt me as much as I hurt myself. They may be trying to make me a victim, but only I can truly succeed in that task.
>
> "I will survive. I will keep cool in this hour of stress. I will not let it block my sleep, I will not let it ruin my stomach. And I will not, by any means, allow it to rot my brain."

Memorize this. Play it over in your mind every time tension seems to overwhelm you. If necessary, keep a tension diary. Mark down where the tension came from, when it occurred, and what happened to the whole situation one week, or one month, or one year after.

You will find, by going back over this diary from time to time, that the situations were not nearly as bad as they seemed to you then. In fact, many of them will look just plain laughable, or trivial to you now.

You can survive. And you can survive without pain!

Other recommendations for chronic tension headaches are these:

1. Apply heat at the first sign of pain, before it becomes a tight band around your head. Wet a towel and wrap it around your head instead. Or take a hot shower, letting the water run on your face and neck and shoulders.

2. Brush your scalp daily to improve blood circulation. This builds the power of your cranial arteries to wash away the pain particles.

3. Swear off alcohol, especially during times of great pressure. It simply makes the pain much greater.

What To Do for Sinus Pain

For a sinus headache, cover your head with a towel, and breathe in the steam from a basin of hot water to which you have added eucalyptus.

However, if the headaches persist, you may have an infection and need an antibiotic. See your doctor.

When To See a Doctor

As you have discovered at some cost, chronic headaches, however excruciating, are rarely life-threatening. This is one reason you are not able to get enough sympathy or support from your family, friends, colleagues, employers or even most doctors.

Therefore, informed trial and error is still the best approach, and can save you a small fortune in doctors' bills.

Still, there are times when continuing headaches may be a sign of organic disease, and a professional opinion should be sought. These times include the following:

1. If you suddenly begin to have them and are over age 40. Headache frequency and intensity usually dwindles as you grow older.

2. If they follow physical exertion or straining. "Exertion" headaches after strenuous sports are fairly common and benign, but you do want to rule out internal head injury.

3. If you have a headache accompanied by a loss of speech or confusion, especially after you have suffered a blow to the head — even one that happened weeks earlier.

4. If you have headaches accompanied by either a very stiff neck or fever.

To Sum Up:
How I Beat The Worst Headache of All —
Recurrent Weekly Migraines

I was a tortured woman for years. I no longer am. I tried doctor after doctor, and they could do nothing but give me pain-killing drugs which quickly lost their effectiveness and had absolutely horrible side effects in my body.

Then I learned to depend on myself, and natural healing. And these are the simple steps that changed my life:

1. I let my mind take care of my head. When the aura begins, I immediately stop what I am doing, and turn to relaxation and visualization. I use the method I have described in detail above. I practiced it over and over again for weeks before it started turning off these headaches as soon as they came up. So should you.

Your imagination may be the greatest weapon ever invented against stress, tension, crisis, disappointment, and all their physical effects, all over your body.

2. I made a simple habit of drinking a cup or two of coffee in the morning. Works wonders for me. Do give it a try.

3. I use a natural healer. In my case, specifically fever-few, ginger and magnesium. Do try this too. But also try the other natural healers I have listed for you in this chapter.

4. In ruling out the headache poison from my diet, I am making sure I do not eat myself into a migraine any more. Therefore, you must test the foods in your life, and eliminate those which are causing you the same trouble.

5. Last of all, I use ice packs whenever another headache shows itself and I am in a place where I can apply them.

That's all it took for me. And I truly believe that something similar will be all it takes for you.

SUMMARY

Possible Headache Triggers

- allergy to food additives, condiments and spices
- anxiety, anger and stress
- appetite suppressants
- changes in barometric pressure or wind conditions
- constipation and bloating
- decongestants
- deflected light into the eyes
- diuretics
- hunger
- lighting that is too dim or too bright
- low blood sugar
- nasal sprays
- oral contraceptives or hormone replacement therapy
- smoking
- spinal misalignments
- temporal mandibular joint (TMJ) problems
- too much headache medication

Foods That May Trigger Headaches

- aged cheese
- alcohol
- avocados
- bananas
- beans
- chocolate
- citrus fruits
- cured meats
- eggplant
- figs
- ice cream
- liver
- nuts
- pickled herring
- salt
- sour cream
- soy sauce
- wheat
- wine

Antidotes To Try

- aspirin, one a day to thin the blood
- calcium
- catnip
- citrus fruits and juices
- coffee (one cup at the start of the day)
- deep breathing and relaxation exercises
- emotional stress evaluation and control
- eucalyptus
- feverfew (bachelor's button)
- heat, then ice packs
- high protein, low sugar diet
- iron
- juice of fresh cabbage, celery, lettuce or green vegetables
- magnesium
- meditation and visualization
- omega-3 fish oil
- peppermint
- powdered or fresh ginger
- raw food, one meal on alternate days
- rosemary
- sage
- seaweed
- vitamin E
- walking and stretching

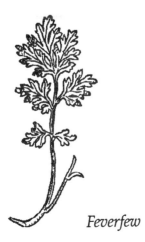

Feverfew

13

Heartburn: Never Again Need You Be A Chronic Heartburn Victim

*Y*ou know the feeling only too well. Out of the blue, suddenly you get an intense, burning sensation that starts behind your breastbone and may reach as far as your throat. Each time this happens, it scares you a little. You probably remember vividly the first time you encountered it, since you may have thought then that you were having a heart attack. And each time it happens, there's always that gnawing suspicion — could this attack be the big one?

You know by now, it certainly wasn't the big one. It was plain, ordinary, common "heartburn." And "heartburn" is a completely misleading term, since the heart has absolutely nothing to do with it. What they call "reflux esophagitis" is the real culprit.

What causes this reflux? Eating something that disagrees with you . . . Continuous overindulgence . . . Eating under stress . . . Or gulping food on the run.

What is the first source of relief you should always try? Bicarbonate of soda or antacid pills. If you are rarely afflicted, they are usually all you need.

What is the first source of relief you should always try? Bicarbonate of soda or antacid pills. If you are rarely afflicted, they are usually all you need.

But what if it has progressed to the stage where almost any meal causes you pain? First, always let your physician rule out an ulcer or other possible causes. He or she will probably tell you that you have a weakness or irregularity of the esophageal sphincter, the ringlike muscle at the bottom of your esophagus. This muscle no longer closes as it should when your stomach is full or under pressure. As a result, food and gastric juices (stomach juices) back up into your esophagus which has no protective lining. And that really hurts!

So you have a weakness inside. But this does not mean you have to become a chronic heartburn sufferer. There are many simple measures you can take to prevent or ease the pain without becoming a slave to pharmaceutical products and their side effects.

Go for Protein, Cut the Fat

Try switching to a high-protein, low-fat diet. According to Mitchell Conn, M.D., and David B. Sachar, M.D., this intake of lean protein will increase esophageal sphincter pressure.

On the other hand, fats decrease the pressure, allowing the unwanted reflux to play havoc.

The number one food to avoid, experts say, is chocolate, because it is nearly all fat and contains caffeine as well.

Herbal Remedies

Ginger has a centuries-old reputation for relief of heartburn and gas. Now we have found that this reputation may indeed have a scientific basis. Ginger contains zingibain which fosters the concentration of digestive enzymes in your saliva and also increases the flow of that saliva. Thus, when digested food enters your stomach, it has far less reason to come up again.

When you prepare your meals, add anise seeds, caraway seeds, dill, mint, sage or summer savory. All give not only delicious flavor, but smooth digestion as well. Try licorice. Millions find it helpful.

Among herbal teas, chamomile seems to be the most highly recommended. Mint tea runs a close second.

Digestive liqueurs, sometimes called bitters, are a common remedy in Europe. Many are brewed by monks. Among the most familiar and available here are Fernet-Branca and Campari. Angostura Bitters in a glass of water gives relief.

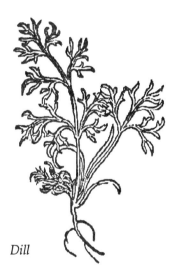

Dill

Banana powder has been said to be an effective antidote for heartburn. So is sipping a teaspoon of apple cider vinegar in half a glass of water. And, because it stimulates saliva in swallowing, sucking on hard candy sometimes works well.

Miscellaneous Do's And Don'ts

- Avoid black pepper and chili pepper.
- Stay away from smoking and drinking coffee. They are poison to your esophagus.
- Be very, very careful about any form of alcohol. This is not an absolute no-no, but should be experimented with

in this way: cut out all alcohol for a few days. Then introduce one glass a day. If this is fine, go back to two glasses a day as I have advised you elsewhere in the book to have as a limit to your daily intake.

Many patients across America have found that their heartburn symptoms almost evaporate just by eliminating or restricting caffeine which is found in chocolate and in many colas, as well as coffee and tea. Oddly enough, decaffeinated coffee also can be irritating, so rule that out, too.

Whole milk should be avoided because of its fat content. As just one example, a real losing combination is having a cigarette while drinking coffee with whole milk, half-and-half or cream.

Citrus juice and tomato juice, paste or sauce may or may not increase your heartburn. Test each one of them individually by cutting each out for a week. See if the heartburn diminishes. If it doesn't, go back to them.

Warning: Do Not Use Antacids For More Than a Month at a Time

Though antacids give harmless relief for the odd bout of heartburn, you really cannot use them to alleviate a chronic condition. Staying on them for more than a month is ill advised, to say nothing of reaching the point where you pop them after every meal.

Antacids that contain aluminum hydroxide and calcium carbonate can cause constipation, while those with magnesium salts may cause diarrhea.

Constant use of antacids containing aluminum hydroxide, either alone or combined with magnesium hydroxide, may interfere with proper absorption of phosphorus, which can weaken your bones.

And those containing sodium bicarbonate (baking soda) or calcium carbonate can lead to an excess of calcium in your body, especially if you consume a lot of dairy products. This may seem good for your bones, but excess calcium can lead to bursitis, calcium (bone) spurs, etc.

Medication and Heartburn

Your doctor may prescribe new drugs which may produce heartburn as a side effect, as has happened to millions. Or they may aggravate your existing attacks. The drugs include: antihistamines, antispasmodics, some heart medications, the progesterone in oral contraceptives, post-menopausal hormone therapy or antibiotics like tetracycline and theophylline for asthma.

Advise your doctor immediately if this happens. He or she will then put you on an alternative drug that does not upset your digestion.

Other Simple Measures You Can Take

❖ Do not wear tight belts or other clothing that constricts your midsection.

❖ If you are overweight, slim down. A flat stomach puts less pressure on your digestive system, which helps curtail reflux.

❖ Try to eat regularly and moderately. Skipping a meal or two and then having large portions at the next meal will overburden your digestive system.

❖ After meals, do not lie down, but stay up and around in order to allow the pull of gravity to work against reflux. This, of course, means giving up late night snacks (except for yogurt, as I mentioned in a previous chapter) which stimulate digestive acids when you are in the worst position — horizontal — to deal with them.

❖ If you are truly a chronic sufferer, elevate the head of your bed with four to six inch blocks. If you do not sleep alone, you might first try banking extra pillows under your head and upper body in a graduated fashion. Do not just place them in a pile at your neck, because you do not want to compound the problem by getting a crick in that poor neck.

In sum, cut out the trigger foods and liquids. Experiment with the natural healers I have given you. Or use a combination of them to do the trick. Eat regularly and moderately. Enjoy your dinners, don't rush them. Then give yourself a little time to smile and relax after every meal. Even better, take a little stroll.

All this should change you from a chronic heartburn sufferer to a person who can be proud of their digestive system.

SUMMARY

Avoid

- alcohol
- black pepper
- carbonated beverages
- chili pepper
- chocolate
- citrus juices
- coffee
- fats
- hot spices
- onions
- smoking
- tomato juice
- tomato paste
- tomato sauce
- whole milk

Watch Out for Reactions from These Medications

- antihistamines
- antispasmodics
- aspirin
- heart medications
- hormone therapy
- oral contraceptives
- tetracycline
- theophylline

Antidotes

- anise seeds
- antacid pills
- apple cider vinegar in water
- banana powder
- betaine hcl with pepsin
- bicarbonate of soda
- bitters in water
- Campari
- caraway seeds
- chamomile tea
- dill
- eat small meals regularly with light snacks in between
- elevate your head and upper body while asleep
- fernet branca
- ginger
- hard candy
- high protein, low-fat diet
- licorice
- lose weight
- mint leaves
- mint tea
- sage
- summer savory
- walk or remain in an upright position for an hour after eating
- wear loose clothing around your waist

14

Hemorrhoids: You Can Conquer Hemorrhoids the Natural Way

$\mathcal{T}$he painful record shows that at one time or another, eight out of ten Americans are beset with hemorrhoids or, as they are more commonly called, "piles." In fact, half of our middle-aged populace sits on them. Ouch!

Yet, with today's natural-healing breakthroughs, none of us — no, not a single one — has to suffer from these itchy, lumpy, sore swellings. Much less should any of us have to undergo expensive surgery for them. There are ample, simple, amazingly effective remedies such as:

* How to make drinking water dissolve hemorrhoids.
* How greens and beans can foil hemorrhoids.
* Do you know how to use rutin for them? Or ox balm? Or horse chestnut tea?
* And last, and perhaps easiest, have you stopped reading while you are on the toilet?

Let's look in more detail at these, and more, and more.

Go for Adam's Ale, and Cut the Salt

When you are thirsty, do you drink nature's own most plentiful healer . . . water? Plain old everyday water.

Most of us — myself included, until I obtained this information — reached instead for a cola or some other soft drink. Colas, in particular, can make hemorrhoids even more itchy . . . so can beer and excessive coffee.

The essential fact is this:

❖ **Fluid intake is essential — especially if the strain of constipation aggravates your hemorrhoids.**

But drinking good old tap water — or if you prefer, bottled brands — or fresh fruit juice are the best, most harmless ways to easily flush out your system.

It's as simple as this. Adequate water — six or eight glasses a day — leads to soft stools. And soft stools pass out of your body without constantly irritating your hemorrhoids.

Hemorrhoids are a result of continuous irritation. Remove the irritation, and you could very easily remove the hemorrhoids themselves.

If your hemorrhoids are not constantly irritated, your body can then act to heal them. To shrink them. To pull them in. To figuratively dissolve them.

But to achieve maximum results, cut way back on your salt intake. Salt makes your body retain fluids, instead of allowing them to cleanse it.

Fight Hemorrhoids With Fiber

Vegetarians have far fewer hemorrhoids because of their high intake of fiber from legumes, including soybeans, vegetables and fruit. This fiber, taken with plenty of fluids, prevents constipation. Constipation is a major cause of your hemorrhoids, due to the pressure it puts on the delicate veins of your anal canal. Fiber bulks your stools and liquid makes them soft and therefore easy to pass. This combination keeps the waste materials moving.

Coarse or unprocessed bran is another excellent source of fiber. Whole wheat, rye or multi-grain bread, bran muffins or cereals such as shredded wheat or oatmeal readily provide it. Brown rice is another option. You can add a tablespoonful or two of bran or wheat germ to baked goods, casseroles, meat-loaf, or soups.

❖ **Caution: if your hemorrhoids are inflamed and your diet has been low in fiber, do not suddenly start bolting that fiber down. Too much fiber too fast can bring on diarrhea, or constipation, which will only aggravate your problem.**

Again, as always, start gently. Then gently increase the amount you take every week. Be sure to drink plenty of fluids.

Rutin Remedies Piles, So Does Citrus Peel

Rutin, a byproduct of milling buckwheat, and citrus peel bioflavonoids are the principle components of a remedy for hemorrhoids recommended by Bernard A.L. Wissmer, M.D.

This Swiss doctor's initial experiment was carried out with 250 patients. It called for a regime of four to six 100 mg capsules daily of trioxyethylrutin in the beginning, followed by two or three every day for three or four more weeks. This bioflavonoid compound, designed to combat capillary fragility (hemorrhoids are inflamed capillaries), gave relief from bleeding and pain in two to five days.

Trioxyethylrutin, also referred to as "P" or vitamin P, is obtainable in capsule form in many health food stores. Foods rich in rutin include rose hips, grapes, plums, black currants, cherries, blackberries and all citrus fruits.

With the citrus fruits, of course, eat the white part of the peel as well.

Heal Hemorrhoids with Ox Balm

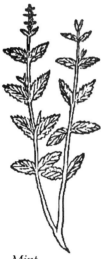

Mint

The classic herb cure for hemorrhoids is ox balm, a member of the mint family also known as horseweed, richweed or stoneroot. In case you are wondering, the folk names with "ox" or "horse" do not mean that the plant comes from, or is used to treat either one. They simply derive from the plant's large size.

Ox balm capsules are available at herbalist's shops. The usual dosage is two 375 mg capsules twice a day with a glass of water during acute flare-ups, or as a preventative daily dose.

An alternative remedy is to place one ounce of the herb in a pint of boiling water. Let it steep and drink half a cup a day.

Look to Horse Chestnut for Help

Extracts or decoctions from the nuts or bark of the horse chestnut tree are also renowned for the treatment of hemorrhoids and other varicose veins. (Do not eat the nuts themselves. While extracts or decoctions are beneficial, eating the nuts can be toxic.)

Herbal Ointments and Suppositories That Ease the Itch

The North American Indians were the first to discover the healing properties of the inner bark of slippery elm. They found that, in contact with water, the mucilage around its fiber swells, providing a soothing salve.

Herbalists often combine five parts slippery elm powder with one part white oak powder in suppository form for hemorrhoids. Or they use yarrow, a plant prized as an astringent and anti-inflammatory agent by the ancient Greeks as well as the Navajos. Yarrow can also be steeped, with an optional teaspoon of goldenseal added, and applied as an ointment.

Here's how to roll your own suppositories:

❖ Mix the powdered herbs with water or vegetable oil. Shape the dough into cylinders 1 to 1 1/2 inches long and 1/2 inch thick. Coat one end with cocoa butter for easy insertion.

❖ If you prefer, just make the suppositories with cocoa butter and herbs. But, if you do, refrigerate them until firm and then bring them to room temperature before you use them.

External Treatments Of Hemorrhoids

Scratching, as you know, only makes matters worse. But bathing soothes. Try to keep your hands away until you can dunk your bottom in warm water. Spread your cheeks so the water bathes the most painful spots.

It is a shame, really, that American plumbing does not include bidets, but you do not have to get into the tub every time. There are plenty of buckets or round plastic basins on the market that are wide and stable enough for fanny-dipping.

For a touch of elegance, treat yourself to hemorrhoid champagne. Put a bottle of witch hazel into a bucket of ice

Witch hazel is particularly effective for the bruised soreness of bleeding hemorrhoids.

and set it beside you. After bathing, use cotton balls soaked with the witch hazel and apply them until they are no longer cold. But apply them to only the external hemorrhoids, please. A few dabs are plenty. Herbalists have believed for a century that witch hazel is particularly effective for the bruised soreness of bleeding hemorrhoids. This is due to the tannic acid of the witch hazel which causes the swollen blood vessels to automatically shrink and contract. A wet teabag will probably have the same effect, because of the tannic acid in tea.

Witch hazel can also be incorporated with glycerin for use as a salve after bathing. Other readily available, recommended emollients include:

- wheat germ oil.
- vitamin E (pierce a soft-gel capsule and apply contents).

Toilet Training

The key here is speed. Get on the toilet and off the toilet. As quick as that.

Do not read or otherwise linger on the toilet. This will only aggravate your condition.

As a lubricating measure, apply petroleum jelly to your rectum to speed transit and protect delicate tissues when hard stools pass.

Some hemorrhoidics find relief from the Clenzone, a small appliance that attaches to your toilet seat and sends a thin stream of water into your anus after a bowel movement.

Or, without resorting to any special device, moisten your toilet paper with warm water and soap to ease wiping. I like to use the packaged, pre-moistened towelettes that are meant for cleansing. They do not fall apart when wet.

Other Piles-Preventive Measures

Do not let your abdomen go to pot. Women are prone to hemorrhoids in the later months of pregnancy because a big belly exerts pressure on the veins and cushions of the rectum. Therefore, unless you are pregnant, when a big belly is natural and needed, keep your mid-section trim.

When you lift anything heavy, protect your hemorrhoids against the strain by stooping instead of bending over. In other words, let your legs do most of the work. Keep your back straight. Do not hold your breath and grunt. Inhale, then exhale and tighten your abdomen muscles as you lift the object.

Hemorrhoids Reabsorbed

I think you will find, without allowing constant irritants or undue pressure and by taking one or more of the steps outlined in this chapter, almost all your hemorrhoids will be effectively reabsorbed.

This holds true even in advanced cases where they have reached the bleeding stage.

However, if your hemorrhoids have not been bleeding for a while and you see a fresh trace of blood, by all means get a doctor's opinion. You want to make sure there is no other problem involved.

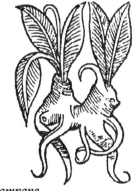

Elecampane

SUMMARY

Remedies

- bioflavonoids (the white membrane and pulp in citrus fruits)
- drink plenty of fruit juices
- eat plenty of vegetables, fruit, whole grains and beans
- horse chestnut extractions (not the nut itself)
- inner bark of the slippery elm salve
- ox balm, also known as horseweed, richweed, or stoneroot
- rutin (a byproduct of milling buckwheat), also found in rose hips, grapes, plums, black currants, cherries, blackberries and citrus fruits
- warm baking soda baths
- water, drink at least a quart daily
- wet teabags used externally
- wheat germ oil, petroleum jelly and vitamin E used externally
- witch hazel used externally
- yarrow, goldenseal, and white oak powder suppositories

Avoid

- beer
- carbonated beverages
- excessive coffee
- salt and foods that are processed
- sitting for long periods on the toilet

15

High Blood Pressure: How To Move Yourself Out of the Danger Range – For Life

By the time you reach 40, your body has taken a lot of abuse. You probably thought your recuperative powers would last forever and you could eat, drink and play to excess without thinking of the future.

Then your doctor tells you that you have high blood pressure. What a shock! You feel alright. There is no reason to believe you have a problem. Why is it so important?

High blood pressure is the silent killer. It can set the stage in your body for heart disease, kidney failure and stroke because of the force it exerts on blood vessels all over your body.

Even worse, no specific symptoms announce its onset. Contrary to popular belief, it does not necessarily make you feel "hyper." Or nervous . . . or hysterical . . . or moody . . . or tense . . . or chronically disturbed. Placid people certainly can have it as well.

That's why it's vital to have your blood pressure checked at least once a year. This is an absolute must. If you don't have high blood pressure, it's a wonderful feeling to know you're okay. If it starts to go up, you can catch it when it's still mild. Even if it has gotten too high — it's been proven that proper diet and exercise will lower it . . . without drugs.

Throw Away Your Salt Shaker

High blood pressure — the medical term for it is "hypertension" — is almost unheard of in primitive societies where salt is not a common additive. Even in our civilized world, salt was a precious commodity for centuries. Not any more! Salt is cheap — too cheap — but all of us pay dearly for using too much of it.

Let's not even mention the phrase "salt sensitive." Some doctors say you should cut down on your salt intake if you are "sensitive" to it. But the best researchers I know now say that every one of us is undoubtedly salt sensitive.

That means salt raises your blood pressure. No doubt about it. No longer any question at all. And therefore the most damaging habit you can have is simply picking up your salt shaker.

Except for one last time. Right now! Put down this book and go into your kitchen. Throw that salt shaker right into the garbage can. And then throw away the large salt container that you use to refill that shaker.

In other words, throw all the salt right out of your house. And keep it out. This one step alone can add 10 to 20 healthy, glowing years to your Second Youth.

Of course, food will taste slightly bland at the beginning. But you'll be astonished, within days, how the food you ate before will seem too salty now.

In a matter of weeks, salt in food will taste bitter and burning to you. You'll wonder how you could ever have tolerated it. Perhaps, for the first time in your life, you'll begin enjoying the natural flavors of all the delicious foods you eat.

Remember, natural Second Youth eating means non-salted eating.

Remember, natural Second Youth eating means non-salted eating.

Salt is a poison. Cut out the salt, and you'll look younger overnight. Bloating will begin to disappear from your body . . . your jitteriness will evaporate . . . and you will begin to feel your arteries flowing freely instead of clogging up. You'll feel a new freedom.

Hidden Salt Is Equally As Bad

Salt contains sodium. Sodium raises your blood pressure. It's as simple at that. Salt makes your body retain fluid, creating a pressure throughout your whole body.

When I look in the mirror each morning, I can tell if I have had salt the day before. There is a distinct puffiness around my eyes. And, the more salt I've had, the heavier my eyelids hang.

Even more alarming is that sodium is also invisible, hidden, lurking in hundreds of products that you eat every day. In fact, the British medical journal *Lancet* estimated that 80 percent of our sodium intake in this country may come from processed foods.

Eighty percent — almost five thousand mg of sodium every single day — coming from foods that we don't even know contain it. Take McDonald's for example. There's more sodium in their apple pie or in their chocolate milkshake than in their regular order of french fries.

So how do you protect yourself against this hidden sodium killer? The rules are simple:

1. Whenever possible, eat fresh, natural foods. If God made them, they don't contain unnatural added salt.

2. If you must use canned products, find low-salt versions, or rinse the salt right off of them. Unless they specifically say "low salt" don't eat them the way they come out of the can.

3. As always, read labels. Check the ingredient list for the words "salt," or "soda," or "sodium," and especially for the symbol *Na*. Buy canned goods or processed foods with the new food labels which specify exactly what percent of your day's sodium intake the food contains.

For example, four dry ounces of Kellogg's *All Bran* contain 1,040 mg of sodium or 43 percent of the recommended daily allowance. And one (6 1/2 ounce) can of *Chicken of the Sea* chunk light tuna in water, drained, contains 994 mg of sodium or 41 percent of your day's recommended sodium allowance.

You can't get processed foods that have no salt or sodium in them. But look for ones that have the lowest amount. And then go back to the natural foods as soon as possible.

4. If you drink water from the tap or buy soft water, know that it also is filled with salt. Again, check the label on the bottled water.

5. Use lemon juice and herbs to flavor your foods. After a week or so they will taste infinitely better.

Herbs and Spices To Choose

The healthiest and best-tasting spices to satisfy your craving for tasty and well-seasoned foods are:

- black, red and white pepper
- cardamon
- dill
- nutmeg
- poppy seed
- powdered mustard
- sage
- turmeric

And the most recommended of all is garlic! Researchers from Bulgaria to Japan as well as France, Germany and Switzerland all report success in treating high blood pressure with this member of the lily family.

Mind Your Minerals

Potassium

You should aim for three times as much potassium as sodium, to avoid fluid retention, swelling and edema, and because diuretics drain the potassium out of your body. And always, as I've said, take a good multi-mineral supplement every day but do not take a separate potassium supplement, except under medical supervision, because it can be slightly toxic.

Food sources for potassium include:

- avocados
- bananas
- beans
- beef
- cantaloupe
- fish
- molasses
- plaintains
- potatoes
- radishes
- raisins
- soybeans
- tomatoes
- wheat germ
- winter squash

Magnesium

Researchers with the Honolulu Heart Program and at the Kobe University School of Medicine in Japan have reported that the higher the magnesium, the lower the blood pressure. Again, your multi-mineral daily pill will give you enough.

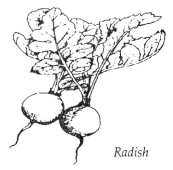

Radish

Food sources for magnesium are:

- almonds
- beans
- Brazil nuts
- brown rice
- cashews
- dark green vegetables
- molasses
- oatmeal
- peanuts
- soybeans
- wheat germ

Be sure to include in your diet: beans, leafy greens, whole grains and lots of fruits and vegetables. Remember that boiling vegetables destroys potassium and magnesium. Steam or stir fry them as I do.

Calcium

Studies conducted at Erasmus University in the Netherlands, at Harvard Medical School, in Oregon and in California indicate that having enough calcium helps keep hypertension under control. Consider that a heavenly bonus because, as you know, calcium is so essential for healthy bones.

I take calcium in supplement form as a part of my daily vitamin/mineral regime. This is the simplest way for me, since I am not sure that I get enough in my diet.

The best natural source for calcium, by far, is low-fat or skim milk. Down your calcium supplement with a skim milk cocktail. Add a little cocoa flavor to satisfy your chocolate craving.

Food sources for calcium are:

- almonds
- Brazil nuts
- broccoli
- cheese
- cottage cheese
- dark green vegetables
- fish
- legumes
- milk
- molasses
- sardines

Fish such as cod, haddock, mackerel, trout, sardines and salmon with bones are exceptionally good sources for calcium.

Fish Oil Foils Hypertension

For years we were told that fatty fish were bad for us, and that we should stick to the leaner swimmers. Then medical science discovered that Eskimos or, for that matter, Mediterraneans also thrive on their local fatty fish catch. Why?

Because such fish as haddock, mackerel, cod, trout, salmon and sardines are rich in omega-3 fatty acids, which help stabilize blood pressure.

You remember your mother telling you that horrible-tasting cod liver oil would make you strong. Well, she was most certainly right, for now there is test after test proving that EPA fish oil — a.k.a. cod liver oil, for example — is good for middle-aged hypertensives.

Significant drops in blood pressure have been obtained by administering from 40 to 50 millimeters per day — that's about four tablespoonfuls. My way of getting this amount is to have three fatty fish meals a week, plus one EPA supplement every three days.

A vegetarian source of EPA is spirulina, an ocean plankton. You can buy it at any health food store. Also note that seaweed is a long standing homeopathic remedy for hypertension. Why not try it, too.

Modify Hypertension With Monosaturates

Experiments by scientists at the University of Kentucky and Stanford University show that consumption of monosaturated fat can cause a significant drop in systolic pressure. Obviously, this will not work if you are still going heavy on the butter or other animal fats. Substitute instead the basic monosaturates olive oil and peanut oil.

Use extra-virgin olive oil with lemon or vinegar on salads and steamed or fast-boiled vegetables. Use it as a base for any number of pasta sauces. Stir-fry vegetables and/or slivered pieces of meat or fish in peanut oil with spices and herbs.

Carbohydrates Calm Hypertension

If you do have high blood pressure, and especially if you feel stressed out much of the time, I highly recommend bread, cereals, corn, crackers, pasta, potatoes, rice and all the other high carbohydrate foods. A diet high in these carbs drives tryptophan into your brain, enabling it to produce the neurotransmitter serotonin which has been shown by recent research to help your brain automatically lower your blood pressure.

Obesity Makes Blood Pressure Soar

One fact science knows without dispute. Hundreds of studies have shown a direct link between excess weight and high blood pressure. Therefore, as you lose that unwanted, burdensome fat, your blood pressure goes down in proportion. And down . . . and down.

What's the best method of blood pressure dieting? Just eat smaller amounts of food more often every day. Instead of three square meals, try six meals plus snacks. Make the meals smaller, and the snacks larger. Never skip a meal, or a snack. Each is equally important.

Cut out the fat. Eat your fill of everything else, especially the natural carbohydrates.

Remember that heavy meals — especially heavy fat meals — send your blood pressure soaring.

On the other hand, light meals send your health soaring.

Lower Your Blood Pressure and Lose Weight With Exercise and Activities!

If your weight and blood pressure are really high, follow your doctor's orders regarding exercise and diet.

But, if your diastolic pressure (the lower number of your reading) is below 104, you can lower that number through exercise and proper diet.

Research has found that 20 to 40 minutes a day of aerobics (exercise that makes the pulse rise to a working level that is specified by your doctor) can reduce your blood pressure to the point where you would not have to take medication.

Each time my blood pressure reads higher than normal, I immediately get on a treadmill or do fast-walking. With headphones emitting music in my ears, the rhythm makes me want to dance on the treadmill. The schedule I try to follow is 20 minutes a day at least three times a week. I am always amazed at how fast my blood pressure drops. And I feel so good because the exercise makes my body more alive.

Activities such as tennis, bicycling, dancing, etc. can be just as effective, and perhaps more fun for you.

Another benefit of all this exercise is weight loss . . . a better appearance . . . and a higher self esteem.

Relaxation Relieves Hypertension

People with high blood pressure are not necessarily high-strung. Yet once it develops, tension and stress seem to aggravate this high blood pressure and move it up notch after notch.

How do you break this deadly spiral?

Simply by rewarding yourself every single day. Life is difficult. You are a hero to survive it every day. For every single day of your life, you deserve such a reward.

Give yourself a break every day, have a good time, or just goof-off for 10 or 15 minutes.

Each one of us has their own way of relaxing. Maybe for you it's a nap. Or looking through *Vogue*. Or gossiping over the phone with an old friend. Or taking off your shoes and wiggling your toes at the world.

Tension and stress seem to aggravate high blood pressure.

Remember, you're never too busy to have this daily break. The world will really take care of itself for those 10 or 15 minutes and worries have a way of evaporating if you leave them alone a little every day. In the next chapter, I'll give you a very easy method of daily meditation which works wonders even for women who say they can't meditate at all.

Treat yourself to a day of luxury at least twice a month or more. Spend a day at the spa. Have a massage . . . a manicure . . . a pedicure . . . get your hair done by a stylist . . . get a facial, etc. Or simply go into a park or sit beside some body of water doing nothing but "taking in the moment." You'll be amazed at the different perspective you will have about your life.

Exercise helps relieve tension too. Sometimes, when I have a full head of steam and muscle knots from tension or stress, I put my body in action. The good endorphins begin to flow and I feel good again.

If you can, get a pet. They are little packages of love. If men had tails like dogs and we taught them how to wag them, there would be no more wars.

If you don't have a pet, borrow one for a few minutes a day. And when that little dog or cat comes to you and settles in your lap, stroke it. You will practically hear your blood pressure cascading down.

People Most at Risk To Develop High Blood Pressure

Those most at risk are blacks, the obese, and women who either have a family history of the problem, a rapid heart beat with no other explanation and/or a high intake of salt or alcohol.

Age is the first factor, starting at 40 and increasing rapidly at 65. Therefore, the further you advance into your Second Youth, the more of these natural tools you must employ to protect yourself against this high blood pressure.

In a few cases, use of birth control pills or underlying medical conditions such as adrenal gland malfunction, kidney disease or a tumor can trigger this high blood pressure. But for the most part, no one knows what causes it. Nor do we have to, since it's now so easy to lower it back toward normal with these Second Youth remedies.

SUMMARY

Ways To Reduce or Prevent High Blood Pressure

- lemon juice is a good substitute for salt
- garlic works wonders for high blood pressure

Use Herbs To Add Flavor and Spice

- black, red and white pepper
- cardamon
- dill
- nutmeg
- poppy seeds
- powdered mustard
- sage
- turmeric

Potassium

- avocados
- bananas
- beans
- beef
- cantaloupe
- fish
- molasses
- plaintains
- potatoes
- radishes
- raisins
- soybeans
- tomatoes
- wheat germ
- winter squash

Magnesium

- almonds
- beans
- brazil nuts
- brown rice
- cashews
- dark green vegetables
- molasses
- oatmeal
- peanuts
- soybeans
- wheat germ

Calcium

- almonds
- brazil nuts
- broccoli
- cheese
- cottage cheese
- dark green vegetables
- fish
- legumes
- milk
- molasses
- sardines

Omega-3 Fatty Acids
- cod liver oil
- cod
- haddock
- mackerel
- salmon
- sardines
- seaweed
- spirulina
- trout

Exercise
- aerobics
- cycles
- stairmaster
- treadmills

Activities
- bicycling
- climbing
- cross-country skiing
- dancing
- fast walking
- rowing
- skating
- swimming
- tennis

A Daily Rest Or Fun Break – Relax And Enjoy Life!

A Day Of Pampering Yourself
- facial
- go to a park
- hair styling
- listen to music
- manicure
- massage
- pedicure
- read a book
- sit by a lake, running brook, the ocean

Meditate Daily

Get A Pet – Or Borrow One for a While

Avoid
- fat
- salt (sodium)
- stress

16

The Immune System: How To Skyrocket The Power of Your Immune System

N o, your immune system alone is not your first line of defense against disease, pain and aging.

Your first line of defense against these three killers is really *the natural foods you use to boost that immune system to a point where disease and pain and aging can't penetrate it.*

Let's look carefully at what your immune system does, and how these natural immune boosters work to keep it in a stage of Second Youth all your life.

Let's leave technical or medical definitions aside. You just don't need them to be in perfect health. What really counts is this — as you grow older, your past habits begin to add up. And the environmental pollution we are all trapped within adds up too.

At the same time, you no longer digest immune-strength-ening foods as efficiently as you once did so you begin taking more and more medication to make up for these deficiencies. But, this medication drains your body's ability to absorb the

You need foods that are the building blocks of your disease fighters

vitamins and minerals needed to make the immune protectors that keep your body young, healthy and strong.

You need certain foods to help you digest other foods more efficiently. You need foods that are rich in anti-aging properties. And you need foods that are the building blocks of your disease fighters.

All of these are immediately available at your local farmers' market, supermarket, or health food store. Many can be grown in your garden or on your window sill. All enable you to draw on nature's bounty directly, in order to build youth and health right back into your aging and damaged body.

In addition, of course, there are the vitamin/mineral supplements I recommend to you in this book. Only the most hidebound members of the medical establishment still question taking them. I certainly rely on them every day. So do most people I know who look terrific at my age, and far older.

Especially if circumstances, including work pressure and business trips, prevent you from having a diet that is balanced and rich in immune-system boosters . . . fill in the gap with supplements.

With daily supplements you can always be sure. You are no longer a victim of chance. You are in control of your future. And that's where you want to be.

Don't Rust Away — Get Your Antioxidants

Do you like cantaloupe, carrots or sweet potatoes? Are you in the habit of drinking orange juice or having half a grapefruit for breakfast? Do you have to remind yourself to buy more olive oil because you are always running out of it? These are sure signs that you are on the right track.

Why? Because such foods are crammed with the antioxidants vitamin A, C and E, and the additional antioxidant beta-carotene.

What exactly do antioxidants do? It sounds very technical, but it's not. The cells in your body simply rust, like a piece of tin left in the air, if you don't protect them. When tin rusts, it turns brown and flaky. When your cells rust, they turn old and weak. Soon the rust crumbles and your cells do too.

Your cells rust because the air inside your body, taken in with your every breath, eats them up. This is called "oxidation."

You can prove this to yourself most dramatically by taking a slice of apple and leaving it on a plate overnight. In the morning, when you look at it again, it will be brown and uneatable. The oxygen in the air of your kitchen has done that to this slice of apple. And, unless you protect every cell in your body, the oxygen in the air inside that body will do the same thing over a longer period of time. And it will do it to your entire body.

Air causes rust. Rust equals age, both inside and outside of your body. It sucks the moisture and lubrication out of your cells.

But now look. Cut another slice of apple and wrap it in clear plastic wrap. Put it in your refrigerator to add a second layer of protection. Then come back to it in the morning and unwrap it. It will still be sweet, moist and delicious. It won't have aged a second.

Antioxidants spread throughout your body and protect your cells against rust.

Why? Because the wrap and the freezing air of the refrigerator kept the active air away from it and it didn't rust. . . or, chemically speaking, burn up.

It was protected against rust, and therefore protected against aging. This is what you have to do with each of the vulnerable cells of your body.

Antioxidants are nature's own plastic wrap. When you eat them or take them in supplement form, they spread throughout your body and protect your cells against rust. The oxygen in your body wants to cause rust, but it can't get close enough to your cells to do this. Therefore, they are protected ... they are no longer continuously damaged and now they have a chance to heal the damage that the former rust has done to them.

Therefore, they can revert back to their youthful stage, or what we have called in this book, *Second Youth*.

Your Two Immune Systems

What you really have protecting your body is not one, but two immune systems.

❖ First, you have the disease-fighting cells in your body which specifically seek out and destroy germs, bacteria, viruses, and poisons.

❖ Second, you have the nutrients and enzymes that you purposely and continually put into your body. They seek out the rust that oxygen carries into your body, and they keep it from damaging or aging your cells.

Two immune systems. Not one. And we are going to strengthen both of them in this chapter.

The Super Vitamins–
The Super Anti-Agers–
The Super Youthifiers!

These foods, herbs, vitamins, minerals and other supplements which follow are cancer protective in that they prevent runaway cell damage. They are anti-heart-disease medicine. They are better for the skin of your face than the most expensive face cream. And they protect against fat on your hips and buttocks better than a five hundred calorie a day starvation diet.

Vitamin A

This vitamin not only preserves night vision and keeps your skin plump, nourished and healthy, but it also acts as a switch to turn on disease-fighting T-cells. According to Susan Smith, Ph.D., research fellow in the Department of Physiology and Biophysics at Harvard Medical School: "With a vitamin A deficiency, this switch doesn't get thrown."

Vitamin A from animal sources, such as butter, beef and beef liver, is high in fat and cholesterol so don't rely on them. Vitamin A supplements, unless used under a doctor's supervision, can be toxic if taken in too high a dosage.

The safest, most effective way I've found to get vitamin A is to use the vitamin A precursor, beta-carotene, which is found in plants. It has no fat and no cholesterol and is converted into vitamin A by your body.

Dozens of studies coming in now indicate that people who eat lots of fruits and vegetables high in beta-carotene have a lower risk of developing cancer of the lung, mouth, throat, stomach, colon, rectum, cervix, skin and esophagus.

All that protection against all those cancers for just a single swallow of a pill, or a few mouthfuls of food!

In addition, current research dramatically shows that beta-carotene's antioxidant properties also thwart heart disease.

Findings of the ongoing Physicians' Health Study indicate that men with cardiovascular problems have only about one-half the risk of stroke, heart attack and death from cardiovascular disease when they are given beta-carotene supplements. All they need is 50 mg every other day, which is roughly equivalent to two cups of cooked carrots.

Beta-carotene is not toxic at high levels when you eat fresh fruits and vegetables, and your bonus is fiber. Paul Lachance, a professor of food science at Rutgers University, affirms that most Americans should consume two to four times more beta-carotene than they do.

Beta-carotene from yellow-orange sources include:

- apricots
- cantaloupe
- carrots
- mangoes
- papaya
- peaches
- persimmons
- pumpkin
- squash
- sweet potatoes/yams

Go for these greens as well:

- Beet greens
- broccoli
- collards
- kale
- spinach
- watercress

Vitamin C

Vitamin C stimulates production of T-cells and interferon which, as the name implies, interferes with the invasion and duplication of bacteria, viruses and cellular debris.

Good food sources are much the same as for beta-carotene — in other words, once you eat one of these foods, you have many healthy immune-system boosters working for you at the same time.

For vitamin C from the vegetable family in particular, add:

- Brussels sprouts
- cabbage
- cauliflower
- parsley
- peppers
- tomatoes

Romanian scientists found that cabbage is one of the most powerful antibody (immune system) stimulants known to men.

From the fruit family, add:

- berries
- citrus fruit
- guava
- pineapple
- sour cherries

And remember that squirting lemon juice on your fruits and vegetables brings out the flavor and ups the vitamin C ration.

Vitamin E

Researchers by the dozen have come to believe that the antioxidant effect of vitamin E is particularly important for strengthening your immune system as you age. There is also ever-accumulating evidence of its preventative value against cancer, and for the treatment of benign breast lumps.

There are not as many food sources for vitamin E as for most other vitamins. Therefore, I would recommend that you take a 400 to 800 I.U. supplement daily. I take 800 myself, but either of those amounts will give you substantial protection against the harm done by free radicals.

The food sources that do exist, nonetheless, are excellent. They include:

- almonds
- cashews
- corn oil
- hazel nuts
- olive oil
- safflower oil
- sesame oil
- walnuts
- wheat germ

I often sprinkle wheat germ on vegetables, add it to soups, or stir it into yogurt which has, of course, other infection-fighting properties of its own.

❖ PERSONAL NOTE: I'll tell you one of my most enjoyable retreats from the busy life I lead.

When I am home alone after a hectic day, I often do not want an elaborate meal. So, I chop, slice, steam or stir fry vegetables, and squeeze the juice of a lemon over them. Or I just make a bowl of mixed salad vinaigrette, then I take it on a tray to the living room, along with a glass of red wine.

Usually, I am barefoot, dressed in leggings and a roomy shirt. I curl up in my very comfortable, cushioned wicker chair in the corner of my living room near my TV set and chomp happily away, with my zapper at hand to change programs at whim.

What Fun! What Relaxation! And each delicious mouthful cleans the body-rust right out of my system.

Another Reason Garlic Is Great for You

As you know by now, garlic has been prized since antiquity for its therapeutic quality, and for what many consider its wonderful flavor. Over the centuries, it has been used for everything, from warding off colds and the plague to alleviating gas pains and chronic bronchitis to ridding the body of intestinal worms and vaginal yeast infections.

Now, modern medical science is proving that the ancients were absolutely right. Garlic contains vitamins A, B^1, B^2 and C, and allicin, or allium oil, which is an inhibitor of vast numbers of fungi and bacteria.

In addition, the most recent research, both here and abroad, has discovered that garlic may stimulate the immune system in general. That means every killer white cell in your body that you rely on for your health. And now, hints are beginning to accumulate about the ability of garlic to block enzymes that foster the runaway production of prostaglandins which promote certain tumors. In fact, studies in China have demonstrated that the more garlic ingested, the less the incidence of stomach cancer.

There is no doubt that garlic can have social drawbacks — it is known as the "stink rose." I suppose that's where the idea of garlic warding off evil spirits came about. Who wants to be around the smell of second-hand garlic?

I, for one, happen to love the taste and aroma of fresh garlic. I do not eat it every day, but am delighted to know that something so inexpensive and available turns out to be so good for my health as well.

When I eat garlic, whether raw or in a dish that is heavily seasoned with it, I make sure to finish my meal with a sprig or two of parsley. It cleanses my mouth and breath. It also helps me maintain my friendships.

Some people do not digest garlic well. Garlicky food makes them ill and they quite rightly shun it.

If you have trouble digesting garlic, or if its odor offends you and your friends, take it in odorless supplements that you can get at your neighborhood health food store.

Mushroom Power

Shiitake mushrooms, now available in many supermarkets, are worth their weight in gold for your health, and they are delicious. One of the first researchers to investigate shiitakes' curative power was an American, Dr. Kenneth Cochran of the University of Michigan, who discovered they contain a substance, lentinan, that stimulates the immune system to fight viruses. Though this is not yet conclusively proven, he found that this substance may stunt the growth of tumors. And now, Japanese research corroborates shiitakes' antiviral effect.

Shiitake mushrooms stimulate the immune system to fight viruses.

Researchers in China, Korea, and Japan have zeroed in on the reishi mushroom as well, due to its long standing popular use for any number of afflictions. In general, scientific evidence regarding this mushroom's immunity-boosting potential is accumulating.

Herbs and Wildflowers That Combat Disease and Aging

The validity of the traditional belief in the preventive and curative power of plants is no longer in question. Here are examples of some native American and Oriental plants whose usage has been proven. Though I cannot vouch for all of them personally, my experience with Siberian ginseng has been illuminating.

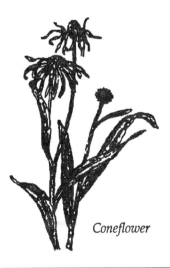

Coneflower

Coneflower (Echinacea)

The Western Plains Indians relied on coneflower for toothaches, enlarged glands, snakebites and other poisonous stings. Now, scientists not only find proof of its external use as an antiseptic, but they have also recognized that extracts of coneflower can stimulate the immune system to alleviate sore throats and the common cold. It does this by increasing the production of antibodies.

Goldenseal

Pioneers quickly adopted this plant from the American Indians as a cure for eye inflammations, to stop bleeding and to enhance the effectiveness of other herbs in herbal remedies. The dried rhizome is thought to be cytotoxic and antibacterial.

As a tea it has been used as a douche for vaginal inflammations. Goldenseal should not be taken without medical supervision because it is poisonous in large doses.

Astragalus or Huang Qi

Recent studies, including those done at the M.D. Anderson Hospital and Tumor Institute, have manifested the immune building faculty of this herb of the pea family. It inhibits pathogens by promoting the growth of antibodies, leukocytes and interferon. It can be obtained in edible or drinkable form at your health food store.

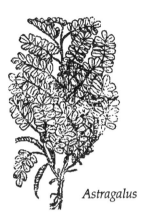

Astragalus

Ginseng

Ginseng is usually classified as an adaptogen. In other words, it does not kill off diseases, but it helps your body overcome them, at least in part by increasing energy and endurance. According to the ancient Indians, Indian ginseng, taken with milk, oil or water for 15 days, restores your weakened body as much as rain does a parched crop. Scientists now believe that this herb promotes what they have named, "state of non-specifically increased resistance."

As for Siberian Ginseng, I first tried it when desperately casting about for a natural remedy for hot flashes due, of course, to the drop in my estrogen level at menopause when my ovaries stopped producing enough of it.

I knew that Siberian Ginseng had long been reputed to fortify the endocrine system so it would take over the manufacture of this vital feminine hormone, but I was still astounded at the results: the hot flashes diminished tremendously.

Combined with the other methods I have given you in this book, I continue to take it in pill form or as a tea, both to forestall post-menopausal problems such as dry, itchy skin and osteoporosis — and because I, indeed, find it energizing. It is a marvelous pick-me-up. Try it today!

One last credential for Siberian Ginseng. A recent double-blind study revealed a considerable increase in overall cellular immunity when an extract of it was administered.

The evidence keeps piling up and up.

Minerals To Mine for Immunity

In recent research, the main emphasis here has been on the revitalizing potential of zinc and selenium alone. If you take a multi-mineral pill every morning, however, you will get sufficient amounts of them, and you'll also get your vital copper, iron and magnesium.

Zinc stimulates the thymus gland, which shrinks as you age, and causes it to create white blood cells that fight off infectious bacteria. Think of it. Over 70 enzymes in your body are dependent upon this zinc. 25 to 50 mg a day is the usual limit so check your one-a-day supplement for its quantity. Excellent food sources are:

- blackstrap molasses
- brewer's or torula yeast
- chicken
- crabmeat
- egg yolks, but no more than three a week
- herring
- lean beef and lamb
- maple syrup
- oats
- oysters
- rye and whole wheat bread
- sesame and sunflower seeds
- soybeans

Selenium

It has taken decades for scientists to recognize the incredible immune-boosting role of selenium. But now research at Colorado State University and elsewhere indicates that selenium enhances both primary and secondary immune responses, and some scientists say the increase is as much as 20 or 30 times. And, adding it to drinking water has been shown to protect test animals from cancer-inducing chemicals.

It doesn't seem that relying on food sources for your selenium is sufficient because the selenium content of soil varies so widely. If the soil is weak, so is the selenium. Therefore, I advocate taking one selenium pill per day in the standard strength sold in most health food stores. The provisional recommended daily allowance for adults is 50-200 mcg and it is sometimes combined with vitamin E.

The Japanese Secret of Lifelong Immunity

For centuries, the Japanese have made seaweed a daily part of their diet. Algae are rich in antioxidants such as beta-carotene, selenium and trace minerals, as well as B-complex, iron and bone-preserving calcium.

Animal studies conducted in Japan and Hawaii show that brown algae, or kelp, such as wakame and kombu — commonly used to wrap the rice for sushi — contain active anti-viral, antibiotic and anti-tumor compounds. Blue-green algae seem to be protective as well.

Not Brown Tea, Please, but Green!

In one of his wry columns for *Newsday*, Robert Reno recounted sitting next to an eminent Japanese oncologist on a 13-hour flight from Tokyo to New York. He was stunned to watch the old boy smoke like a chimney, wade in cognac, and then go jauntily off to deliver a lecture on cancer.

How did this Japanese gentleman do it? he wondered. What secret of good health and longevity did he possess? Shortly thereafter, several medical reports in the press caught Reno's attention. One concerned green tea which is made from unfermented green leaves and is immensely popular in Japan and many parts of China. It alone might well be a reason why Orientals who smoke heavily have nowhere near the lung cancer rates of the Americans who smoke.

Indeed, scientists at the National Cancer Research Center in Tokyo believe it can inhibit the growth of cancer cells.

Research presented at the first international symposium on the health effects of green tea would also intimate that it lowers blood pressure and cholesterol as well.

This news hit within days of the Harvard School of Public Health study, which concluded that regular consumption of alcohol staves off dying from a heart attack. Two ounces a day reduces your chances of a heart attack by 25 percent, and three ounces by 50 percent.

"Swearing off bacon and eggs, stuffing yourself with oat bran and blood thinners, won't give you these sort of figures," the columnist gleefully noted. And he added that this reduction was far more dramatic than that obtained by "a lot of the slop turned out by the pharmaceutical companies that costs a fortune and has ghastly side effects that make you wish you were dead anyway."

What Vitamin/Mineral Supplements To Consider And Why!

If you take medication, you need these supplements to offset the depletion of vitamins and minerals.

I have no doubt that the best way to obtain the nutrients for good health is from food; but for a maximum boost to your immune system, take supplements as well. If you take them as you grow older, you combat the cumulative effect of environmental pollution . . . you let your body repair itself from past or present bad habits and you compensate for digesting less efficiently. Also, if you take medication, you need these supplements to offset the depletion of vitamins and minerals that medication causes.

This has been proven by medical science over and over again. As just one example, in the 1992 Canadian study authored by Dr. Ranjit Kumar Chandra, people 65 years and older were given a capsule containing modest daily amounts of a broad spectrum of vitamins, minerals and other supplements.

When compared to a test group, those given the supplements had considerably — that is *considerably* — fewer infections and stronger immune defenses. The study lasted for a full year and involved 96 men and women.

The18 ingredients in the capsule were:

- vitamin A
- vitamins B^6 and B^{12}
- vitamins C, D and E
- beta-carotene
- calcium
- copper
- iodine
- iron

- folate
- magnesium
- niacin
- riboflavin
- thiamine (B^1)
- selenium
- zinc

Interestingly enough, the amount of vitamin A was roughly half the daily allowance recommended by Canadian and American health authorities, whereas the amounts of beta-carotene and vitamin E were three to four times higher.

Regarding readily available, commercial multi-vitamin and mineral pills, *Theragran-M* is said to have one of the best balances. The one I take offers much the same formula, but is a New York drugstore chain brand that costs less. As always, shop around to get the most for your money. Sometimes the generic brand in a health food store is cheaper and as my surgeon husband always said, "vitamin C is vitamin C regardless where it comes from."

When compared to a test group, those given the supplements had considerably fewer infections and stronger immune defenses.

This is my daily regime. To increase absorption, some of the supplements are taken in a smaller quantity twice a day, rather than all at once.

Morning

- one high potency vitamin/mineral pill
- one super B-complex pill
- selene (selenium) with vitamin E and Lecithin
- vitamin C, 1500 mg. with time release
- vitamin E, 400 I.U.
- microcrystalline calcium, 500 mg

Night

- vitamin C, 1500 mg. with time release
- vitamin E, 400 I.U.
- microcrystalline calcium, 1000 mg

I want to emphasize that this is a moderate supplement list. In fact, if you are a health enthusiast as I am, it may be too moderate for you. In that case, I offer the list of supplements found by Dr. William H. Lee, one of the nation's leading nutritionists, that has been shown by the most recent research to protect against the damage of free radicals.

- vitamin C – up to 5,000 mg daily
- vitamin B[6] – up to 100 mg daily
- vitamin E – up to 400 I.U. daily
- pantothenate (B[5]) – up to 100 mg. daily
- niacin – up to 100 mg daily
- vitamin A – up to 20,000 I.U. daily
- paba – up to 100 mg daily
- folic acid – up to 400 mcg daily

- Selenium – up to 200 mcg. daily
- zinc – up to 50 mg daily
- magnesium – up to 500 mg daily
- bioflavonoids – up to 250 mg daily
- beta-carotene – up to 25,000 I.U. daily
- L-cysteine – up to 250 mg daily
- L-methionine – up to 50 mg daily

Again, let me stress the fact that, although I recommend taking these supplements every day, they do not and cannot replace the natural, delicious, filling and youthifying foods that contain the same vitamins and minerals. Both supplements and foods interact. One reinforces the other. Feast your way to *Second Youth*. But take supplements as well to guarantee that you have the protection to get there in the surest way possible.

SUMMARY

Antioxidants (from foods below or as supplements)

- beta-carotene
- bioflavonoids
- folic acid
- L-cysteine
- L-methionine
- PABA
- pantothenate
- vitamin A
- vitamin B^6
- vitamin B^{12}
- vitamin C
- vitamin D
- vitamin E

Minerals To Take as Supplements

- calcium
- copper
- folate
- iodine
- iron
- magnesium
- niacin
- riboflavin
- selenium
- thiamine
- zinc

Foods To Eat

- almonds
- apricots
- beet greens
- berries
- broccoli
- brussels sprouts
- cabbage
- cantaloupe
- carrots
- cashew nuts
- cauliflower
- citrus fruits
- collard greens
- corn oil
- garlic
- grapefruit
- guava
- hazel nuts
- kale
- mangoes
- olive oil
- oranges
- papaya
- parsley
- peaches
- peppers
- persimmons
- pineapple
- pumpkin
- reishi mushrooms
- safflower oil
- sesame oil
- shiitake mushrooms
- sour cherries
- spinach
- squash
- sweet potatoes
- sweet potatoes/yams
- tomatoes
- walnuts
- watercress
- wheat germ

Foods that Contain the Listed Minerals

- blackstrap molasses
- blue-green algae
- brewer's or torula yeast
- brown algae/kelp (wakame and kombu)
- chicken
- crabmeat
- egg yolks
- green tea
- herring
- lean beef & lamb
- maple syrup
- oats
- oysters
- rye bread
- seaweed
- sesame and sunflower seeds
- soybeans
- whole wheat bread

Herbs and Plants

- astragalus/huang qi
- coneflower
- ginseng
- goldenseal

17

Osteoporosis: How To Build Second Youth Bones

$\mathcal{I}$ love to dance, don't you? Especially in the open air, at night, under a summer moon. With someone I love very much, to slow, smooth, romantic music.

I love to be held in his arms, gliding across the floor till the wee hours of the morning. To feel myself floating with my feet barely touching the floor. To easily bend when he dips me backwards at the end of each number. Or when he sends my body out in a rhumba, and I circle slowly and seductively around him. Or when we look away from each other, and discover that the rest of the people are sitting exhausted at the tables around us.

I also love to pick up my granddaughter. To hold her in the air above my head, and see her huge smile gleaming down at me. Or chase her on my hands and knees, playing hide and seek. Or dance her to sleep on my shoulder. I love to be able to do my own housework, when I want everything especially clean. Or carry my own bags easily from the car to a waiting plane. Or hit a strong ball over the net in tennis or volleyball. Or be able to drive almost as far as my male partner in a golf foursome.

I show absolutely no bone loss at 59 years of age.

I am 59 years old, and have the kind of Second Youth bones, muscles, and zest for life that allow me all these thrills every day of my life.

There's no reason in the world why you can't have them, too.

My Heredity

My doctor says I show absolutely no bone loss at 59 years of age. Of course, much of this is due to the fact that I come from sturdy Welsh and Slavic stock that gave me strong bones. But I know from my grandmother and my aunts that even these sturdy-at-birth bones can turn fragile at 40 or 50, if we don't take care of them.

One other fact you should know. Strong-framed as I turned out to be, I had rickets as a child. Why? Because my father had left us when I was very young and my mother could not afford enough for us to eat. It could have crippled me, but I overcame it. All my life, I've been making up for that threat. And that is why I, almost better than anyone I know, am so acutely aware of the danger of over-40 bones.

Estrogen Loss Equals
Loss of Strength in Your Bones

Let's review again the orthodox medical view of fragile bones, which they call osteoporosis. Why do your bones grow weak as you grow older? Very simple. As you age, the production of estrogen by your body slows down. And when you go through menopause, it completely stops.

What effect does this have on your bones? Again, the answer is simple. Estrogen slows the breakdown of your bones. Like any other organ of your body, the older you become, the faster this breakdown occurs.

Your skin develops wrinkles, your hair turns grey, and the strength of your bones drains out of your body. As a young woman, when you were producing enough of this natural hormone, the strength remained in those bones. Now, month after month, it just drains out and they become porous and brittle.

Doctors recognize fully that this is a tragic situation for you. Weak bones are fragile bones, and fragile bones can easily shatter. One fragile step, one strain too much and that bone can snap and you can be crippled for life.

Or — to be more correct — you *could have been* crippled for life. Because the doctor will now recommend estrogen replacement therapy to prevent such crippling weakness. And he or she will recommend estrogen replacement therapy, knowing full well that it might increase the risk of cancer in the latter half of your life. (Although research recently reports that estrogen may prevent certain cancers in post-menopausal women, there has not been any unqualified agreement among researchers that estrogen supplements are risk-free.)

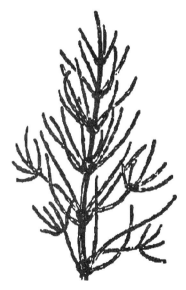

In fact, there have certainly been cases, when a women seems to be breezing through menopause, showing no outward signs of fragile bones, in which the doctor still recommends the estrogen replacement therapy . . . just to be "safe."

This, to my mind, is unacceptable. Estrogen replacement therapy is not for me. I have tried several types of prescribed estrogen and progestin replacements to alleviate the undesirable effects of menopause. They were miserable failures. I have found a far better way.

Horsetail

Plant and herb estrogens unlock the heavenly gate to Second Youth

That way is the natural healing, natural prevention in nature's supply of plant and herb estrogen. I promise you: they make your bones as strong as a horse's.

Remember, Mother Nature prepares for exactly this kind of emergency. If your body no longer gives you the estrogen you need, she supplies the plants and herbs from every continent in the world to give you that supply, instead.

In other words, during and after menopause, plant estrogens take the place of human estrogens. Go back now to the chapter on Young Woman's Hormones, and review everything I've said about these plant and herb estrogens.

Take them, not only for youth, but strength. Take them every day. Without fail. Religiously. For they are the main key that unlocks the heavenly gate for you to Second Youth.

Now you have your supplementary estrogen supply. Let's go on to the other natural remedies for fragile bones.

How To Take the Right Kind of Calcium To Rebuild Second Youth Bones

Calcium is the main building block of bone. Most experts agree that a minimum of 800 mg daily is needed, but many go beyond that, and advise 1500 mg a day. I agree. You need mega-doses of calcium. And I echo their belief that these 1500 milligrams should come primarily from natural sources. I will tell you the richest sources of calcium and I will tell you how to keep it in your bones.

What are the best natural sources? Milk, certainly is the most natural source. But, of course, it also has, for many people, its disadvantages.

Lactose Intolerance

This simply means that milk grievously upsets the stomachs of many people. Therefore, they cannot take it, even in small amounts in commercially prepared foods. Therefore, milk is out for them.

Other people dislike skim milk, which is the healthiest form. Whole milk simply has too much fat, and I advise strongly against it. Try one percent fat milk. Or even two percent milk. Or any of the other types where the fat is drained off before you ever touch it with your lips. I've found it to be especially satisfying with your morning cereal — which I consider essential. But, if you miss the sweetness of whole milk, I would advise a little honey, sugar, or even a little of the so-called natural sweeteners which, in this limited amount, have not proved to be damaging to your health in any way.

The last drawback with milk is that you must drink a large, large amount of it every day to gain the quantity of calcium you need. For example, a glass of milk provides about 275 mg. Therefore, you would have to drink a quart a day to supply your calcium need.

Why not look into skim/no-fat yogurt? Eight ounces of it gives you 450 mg of calcium. And it is much more easily digested than milk.

Or, among other dairy products, cheese is a ready source. But, here again, you must be aware of the saturated fat content in most cheeses. I would suggest that you try low fat, or nonfat cheeses — most of which are thoroughly tasteless — but you may find one or two that please you, at least alternately.

Non-Dairy Sources of Calcium

I love fish and seafood, and more and more medical evidence piles up every day that it is one of the best foods of any sort you can eat, for many reasons. Here are some calcium-loaded fish and seafood choices that you should include at least a few times every week. Sardines and salmon (canned, with bones) . . . mussels . . . oysters . . . and shrimp.

Also seaweed. Kelp and agar are especially rich in calcium. There is no doubt that they both are an acquired taste, but certainly try them. And you might also want to try kelp tablets.

Soybean products not only contain calcium, but act like estrogen to keep it in your bones.

The best calcium vegetables are beet and collard greens. Among legumes, don't just stick to chickpeas, pinto and navy beans, but aim for soybeans also. Most of these have at least a dozen health advantages.

Let's look into that soybean opportunity a little more deeply. In America, we think that dairy products are crucial to building and preserving strong bones. But in the Far East, especially in China and Japan, dairy products are almost completely discriminated against.

What does this mean? That dairy products are not essential and even unnecessary. Oriental women, for example, suffer far less from osteoporosis than Caucasian women. Recent medical research indicates that it is soybeans which do the job for them. Perhaps that's why soybeans are dubbed the "meat" of the Orient. Soybean products — tofu, soy flour, sauce, etc. — not only contain calcium, but they act like estrogen to keep that calcium in your bones.

Again, eat a lot of them. You'll bless the day you began.

Free Calcium

Do you live in an area where the water is hard? Do you sometimes grumble about the white deposit on your pots and pans? Has your tea kettle become so encrusted inside that it's heavy even before you fill it with water?

Well, stop grumbling, and unless your hands are arthritic, hang on to that precious old kettle. For it is giving you free calcium without your even trying. It isn't much, but it all adds up.

So have your hot water system softened if it makes your laundering easier. But keep that cold water hard.

Horsetail To Make Your Bones As Strong as a Horse's

For an extra bonus, boil water in that kettle to make horsetail tea. When you steep the leaves of this rushlike, flowerless plant, you get a brew very rich in calcium, and also silica (a more easily absorbed form of silicon). Both, of course, build strong bones.

How To Take Calcium Supplements

In addition to my natural sources, I do, most certainly, take calcium supplements. But I want to stress right at the beginning of my discussion about them, that they really should be only a second source of calcium in your life, not the primary source. Think of them as backup and booster.

As always, foods and herbs should give you the bulk of the Second Youth nutrients and healers you need.

In the extensive research I've done, the supplement most recommended is calcium carbonate combined with vitamin D. I take it in microcrystalline pills, 500 mg each. And I take one with each meal, which gives me a total of 1500 mg daily.

If you can do it, these three doses a day are the most effective way to distribute calcium's benefits throughout your body. But, if for any reason you can't, do make sure that you get at least one pill a day.

The last thing you want is to pay your good money for calcium foods and supplements, and then have it disappear down the toilet. It will never happen to you again if you follow a simple test.

According to Paul Miller, M.D., associate clinical professor of medicine at the University of Colorado Health Sciences Center School of Medicine in Denver, here is an excellent way to test a calcium supplement for absorption by your body.

Take two tablets from the bottle, and drop them in about six ounces of vinegar. Wait for half an hour, stirring the mixture occasionally. If at the end of the half hour they have not broken up into small pieces, they probably will not dissolve in your stomach. Therefore, change brands at once and test each new supply of calcium you buy.

Each calcium supplement you take should be downed with a full glass of water. I would suggest that you take at least 500 mg a day, and preferably 1,000 mg. However, start with 500 mg. And, if you have a family history of kidney stones, for goodness sake check with your doctor before taking them.

I would not take your calcium in antacids, even if they say calcium carbonate on their label. This is because they make the acid/base balance of the stomach and intestines more alkaline. And this, in turn, reduces the amount of calcium your body can absorb. Therefore, taking your calcium in an antacid base works against itself.

Also, above all, avoid antacids that are aluminum based. First of all, they actually deplete calcium. And second, the aluminum in them has definitely been linked to Alzheimer's disease.

Vitamins that Help Your Body Pour the Calcium Into Your Bones

Your goal is not just to swallow the calcium, but to have it get deeply into the structure of your bones. This means it must be easily digested by your stomach, and then flow right through your bloodstream into the bones themselves. The last thing you want is to pay good money for calcium rich foods and supplements, and then have it disappear down the toilet.

The best calcium helper vitamins are A, B^6, C, D and K. They are the vitamin storers.

Let's look at them one by one.

Vitamin A

One of the least known properties of vitamin A is its ability to help remove old bone cells and form new ones. Out with the old, in with the new — isn't that the main theme of your Second Youth program?

The natural sources of vitamin A include:

- carrots
- dark green, leafy vege-
  tables and herbs, such
  as collard and turnip
  greens, kale, parsley
  and watercress
- liver
- red pepper
- squash
- yams

Vitamin B^6 seems to both strengthen connective tissue and neutralize homocysteine, a harmful substance now found to contribute to osteoporosis.

Vitamin B^6

Natural sources of vitamin B^6 include:

- alfalfa sprouts
- brewer's yeast
- brown rice
- legumes such as lentils
  and soybeans
- rye
- sunflower seeds
- whole wheat

Vitamin C

Vitamin C plays a dual supportive role. First, it acts as an escort system for the calcium to insure that it arrives where it's needed in the bones. And second, it speeds up the production of collagen, a glue-like substance that makes cells stick together in bones as well as in soft tissue.

Good sources of vitamin C are:

- acerola cherries
- black currants
- citrus fruits
- green peppers
- guavas
- parsley
- persimmons
- rose hips
- strawberries
- tomatoes
- watercress

Vitamin D

Older women just don't get enough vitamin D from natural sources

Vitamin D enables your small intestine to absorb larger and larger amounts of calcium. It is also the one vitamin which you can have without spending a cent. Why? Because being in the sun can give you just about what you need every day, at least in the summer.

Now I know that most doctors have reminded us, over and over again in the recent years, about the link between overexposure to the sun and skin cancer. And they are absolutely right, at least as far as overexposure is concerned. It is always bad for you, and you should never do it.

But there is a way around this dilemma. In the summer it is good for you to get out in the sun — *if* you choose only the early morning hours (between 7 and 10 a.m.), and the late afternoon hours (between 4 and 6 or later).

The trick here is to go out in the sun only when your shadow is as long as your body. Limit your exposure from half an hour to an hour. Walk if you can. That way, you'll get, not only calcium-absorbing vitamin D, but also bone-strengthening exercise for your entire body.

Food sources for vitamin D are:

- butter
- cold-water fish
- egg yolks
- meat, especially organ meats such as liver

I can see you worrying now about your cholesterol but, when consumed with moderation, these meats are fine.

Incidentally, studies indicate that older women just don't get enough vitamin D from natural sources, perhaps because it isn't metabolized as well with age. So this is one vitamin you should make sure you get in supplement form. I suggest 400 mg every other day. Not every single day, but every other.

In his booklet, *Beat Osteoporosis For Life*, Dr. Stephen Langer rates vitamin K as a star performer in maintaining strong, healthy bones. He explains that this vitamin enables your bones to synthesize osteocalcin, which is a protein base to which calcium attaches in order to build new bones.

Vitamin K

Natural sources of vitamin K are:

- alfalfa
- Brussels sprouts
- cheeses such as camembert and cheddar
- oats
- soybeans
- soy lecithin

Magnesium

Calcium alone does not do the complete job.

In addition to calcium, you must also have phosphorus, and magnesium.

I don't think you have to concentrate too avidly upon phosphorus, since it is found in most foods, and many food additives. Assume, therefore — especially if you take a good multi-mineral supplement every day — that your supply of phosphorus will be adequate.

Magnesium, however, is a completely different story. On average, American women get only about one-half to three-quarters of the magnesium they should have every day. This means that you've got to eat more magnesium-rich foods, and, again, take that multi-mineral supplement every day.

Good food sources of magnesium are:

- almonds and almond butter
- Brazil nuts
- cashew nuts
- dark green and leafy vegetables
- dried fruits
- filberts
- legumes
- pecans
- sesame and sunflower seeds
- walnuts
- whole grains

Helpful Trace Minerals

The latest medical discoveries have shown that it would be very wise for you to also insure adequate intake of what are called trace minerals — especially manganese (not to be confused with magnesium) and boron.

Manganese

Foods and nutrients containing manganese include:

- barley
- buckwheat
- cloves
- ginger
- ginseng
- legumes
- nuts
- oats
- sunflower seeds
- tea leaves
- whole wheat

Boron

As for boron, very little is really found in food, but, fortunately, very little is needed. Sources are:

- apples
- dates
- honeynuts
- legumes
- pears

Three-milligram supplements are available in tablet form.

I want to point out that there is huge promise in this tiny trace mineral. A recent U.S. Department of Agriculture study showed that, by taking three milligrams of boron daily, a group of post-menopausal women not only lost less strong-bone minerals, but also doubled their blood level of estrogen. Wow!

> Let me add, however, that you should not take more than three milligrams a day. Three milligrams a day . . . and that's it.

Now Let's Break Those Habits
That Break Down Your Bones

Heavy drinking leeches calcium right out of your bones. This occurs in men as well as women, and, though they suffer later, by middle age male alcoholics are also highly prone to those brittle bones.

One drink a day is great. I recommend it highly. It relaxes you and, if taken at dinnertime, separates the night's pleasures from the day's work.

Doctors now feel that even two drinks a day may be beneficial for your heart, for instance. But I prefer the one drink a day, because two tend to fuzz my mind a little.

Remember, we're talking about one bottle of beer, or one glass of wine, or one shot glass full of stronger drinks. That's all!

The caffeine in coffee is another maker of brittle bones, if you drink it all day. But certainly one cup or two during the day will not hurt. I love my morning cup which gets me started with a bang. And I love my early afternoon cup equally as much, to pick me up and keep me going at the same high pitch of energy.

But I do pride myself on being smart enough not to drink coffee after 4 PM. After that, it not only blocks sleep, but it also blocks the bone restorers that your entire body so desperately needs.

Smoking has a hundred different ways to cripple and kill you.

As for smoking, if you haven't already given that up, do so at once! Smoking has a hundred different ways to cripple and kill you. It is the incarnation of Dracula for every one of us. You've probably heard this a hundred times, but do you know that your estrogen level is lowered with every cigarette.

You just can't smoke and attain Second Youth.

Also be aware that salt impedes your body's ability to use calcium. As do animal fats. As do foods rich in oxalic acid — chard, chocolate, rhubarb and spinach.

My champion contender for the most dangerous substance of all is aluminum which you can unknowingly absorb
from aluminum cookware, baking soda, certain deodorants
and antacids.

Aluminum weakens your bones and poisons your brain.
Not just osteoporosis, but also Alzheimer's, may certainly be
in the future of those who are contaminating themselves with
this metal.

Read labels. Buy no deodorant or antacid that has the
word aluminum anywhere in their labels. Protect yourself.
Your life depends on it!

Dracula Drugs

Here they are:

- antibiotics
- anti-depressants
- barbiturates
- chemotherapeutic drugs
- corticosteroids
- cholesterol-reducing drugs
- diuretics
- laxatives.

All have been proved to suck calcium from your bones.
Obviously, when your doctor prescribes one of them, you must
follow his or her recommendation. But, if that happens, compensate for their damage by the means I have given you above.

Even better, see if you can't — slowly, over time, with the
knowledge and consent of your doctor — substitute some of
the natural healers in this book. They don't have any side
effects. They don't cause the damage the prescription drugs do.

There is no reason at all for you to suffer from osteoporosis. Doctors have conclusively proved this over the past few
years. Simply follow the instructions given you in this chapter, and you'll run, play, and dance for the rest of your Second
Youth life.

To sum up: *you can have the bones of a young woman for your first hundred years.*

SUMMARY

Foods To Eat

- calcium
- agar
- chickpeas
- comfrey
- cottage cheese
- horsetail tea
- kelp
- lactose-free milk
- low fat cheese
- mussels
- navy beans
- oysters
- pinto beans
- salmon
- sardines
- seaweed
- skim or low fat milk
- soybeans
- yogurt

Vitamin A

- carrots
- dark green leafy vegetables
- liver
- parsley
- red pepper
- squash
- watercress

Vitamin B^6

- alfalfa sprouts
- brewer's yeast
- brown rice
- lentils
- rye
- soybeans
- sunflower seeds
- whole wheat

Vitamin C

- acerola cherries
- black currants
- citrus fruits
- green peppers
- guavas
- parsley
- persimmons
- rose hips
- strawberries
- tomatoes
- watercress

Vitamin D

- butter
- cold-water fish
- egg yolks
- meat
- organ meats, such as liver

Vitamin K

- alfalfa
- Brussels sprouts
- oats
- soybeans
- soy lecithin
- camembert cheese
- cheddar cheese

Magnesium

- almonds and almond butter
- brazil nuts
- cashew nuts
- dark green and leafy vegetables
- dried fruits
- filberts
- legumes
- pecans
- sesame and sunflower seeds
- walnuts
- whole grains

Manganese

- barley
- buckwheat
- cloves
- ginger
- ginseng
- legumes
- nuts
- oats
- sunflower seeds
- tea leaves
- whole wheat

Boron

- apples
- dates
- honeynuts
- legumes
- pears

Supplements

- boron
- calcium carbonate with vitamin D
- magnesium
- manganese
- phosphorus
- vitamin A
- vitamin B^6
- vitamin C
- vitamin K

Caution! Avoid!

- animal fats
- antacids with aluminum
- anti-depressants
- antibiotics
- barbiturates
- calcium supplements in an antacid base
- chemotherapeutic drugs
- cholesterol-reducing drugs
- corticosteroids
- diuretics
- laxatives
- oxalic acid, found in chocolate, chard, rhubarb and spinach
- products that have aluminum in them
- salt
- smoking
- too much alcohol
- too much caffeine

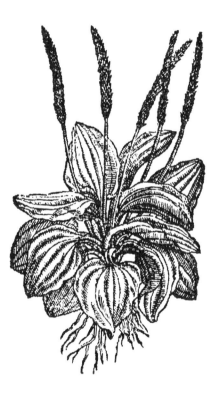

18

Ulcers: Why Your Second Youth Will Never Be Marred By An Ulcer

A bout one person in ten in this country will suffer from an ulcer. If you don't have one now, don't bother to read this chapter. The instructions in the rest of this book will protect you against one.

But if you do have an ulcer, the following information should be invaluable to you.

You Can Cure Most Ulcers Quickly By Yourself

Most ulcers heal within two to six weeks with whatever medication is prescribed to neutralize stomach acidity, and/or coat the lining of the ulcer crater. For that matter, Australian researcher Barry Marshall, M.D. points out that you probably already have the next best thing to a cure in your medicine cabinet: *Pepto-Bismol*.

However, if you are ulcer prone, why suffer the pain? Why resort to medication when all you need to prevent ulcers is to know what foods and supplements to emphasize, and to pace the way you eat.

The Way You Eat Can Make All The Difference

While eating seems to act as a buffer to alleviate the pain of duodenal ulcers, it stimulates gastric secretions which may intensify gastric ulcers. With either type, however, researchers now recommend well-spaced, regular meals of moderate size rather than the old-fashioned regimen of frequent, small meals. Late evening snacks, in particular, should be avoided, in order to avoid being wakened by pain during sleep.

Even more important, bland diets are no longer the order of the day, unless you have complications. You may be advised not to eat red chili peppers, because they stimulate gastric secretions. Yet, according to research published in the British medical journal, *Lancet*, no evidence of clinical ill effects exists for them. And other spicy foods are also not off limits, if you enjoy them.

The same goes for high fiber foods which can be quite helpful because they soothe the stomach lining. The only exceptions would be those with abrasive roughage, such as nuts, popcorn and seeds.

Coffee does not cause ulcers. Still, you should cut way down on your consumption of coffee, including decaf, and also alcohol, because they do stimulate acidic digestive juices. Why not have them exclusively with meals?

Peel A Plantain

Plantains have long been used in India as a folk remedy for peptic ulcers. British and Indian researchers have found valid reasons for this: plantains contain a substance that works much the same way as the anti-ulcer drug carbenoxolone, but without the unwanted side effects. First, they strengthen the gastrointestinal wall, and then they induce healing.

The most powerful form is a powder made from unripe, green plantains. For example, Indian bread made with flour ground from green plantains is highly effective. Ripe plantains apparently do not work as well, but the unripe fruit itself, whether boiled, fried or baked, also seems to cure.

Where do you find them? In any grocery store or supermarket frequented by Hispanic-Americans.

Find Relief in the Cabbage Patch

As long ago as 1940, Dr. Garnett Cheney, a professor at the Stanford University School of Medicine, announced that raw cabbage or, better still, cabbage juice helps heal ulcers. Tests with patients and prisoners at San Quentin had corroborated his hunch. Since then, German, Hungarian and Indian researchers have proved the same conclusion. Why? Because cabbage contains gefarnate, a substance used in anti-ulcer drugs.

Spring or summer cabbage is best. You should mash it up fine in a blender to get the highest concentration, and use that for your liquid intake of six to eight glasses per day.

And, of course, eating cabbage raw or cooked is so good for your health in so many ways that you should always make it a side dish at two or three of your dinners every week.

Eating cabbage raw or cooked is good for your health in so many ways. Make it a side dish at two or three dinners every week.

Zinc Supplements Cure Ulcers

Recently, Dr. Donald J. Frommer of the Department of Gastroenterology at Prince of Wales Hospital in Sydney, discovered that 90 to 150 milligrams of zinc sulfate administered to ulcer patients resulted in a healing rate three times faster than those not so treated. Ask your doctor about this. Check out this rather high dosage of daily zinc.

> Research shows that essential fatty acids increase prosta-glandins, which prevent ulcerations in general. Why not add a daily pill of EPA's to your diet?

And also, of course, eat zinc-rich food sources such as crabmeat, oysters, lean beef or pork, lamb, dark turkey meat and cowpeas.

Should You Use Milk?

Probably not. The cons seem to balance out the pros. And, since you have so many more unabashedly beneficial healing agents in this chapter, why not simply forego milk and use them?

Healing Nutrients and Herbalists' Remedies

Vitamins A, E, and B complex are extremely protective.

Research has also shown that essential fatty acids increase prostaglandins which have been shown to prevent ulcerations in general. Why not, therefore, add a daily pill of EPA's to your diet.

Classic Western herbalist remedies include alfalfa and licorice root, the latter either sucked on or brewed for tea. However, if you have high blood pressure, do not use licorice because it can elevate blood pressure.

Indians use ashwagandha to slash the number of gastric ulcer attacks. And in Japan, nori, the type of seaweed in which sushi is usually wrapped, is strongly believed to contain an anti-ulcer substance.

It is essential, of course, to see your doctor. Do you really have an ulcer or is it just heartburn or dyspepsia? All three can cause that gnawing, burning pain in your stomach or upper middle abdomen shortly after eating, or in the middle of the night.

To add to this confusion, if you take an over-the-counter antacid, as you would for indigestion, you will often help relieve ulcer pains as well.

The big problem is that if you leave the ulcer unrecognized, it could lead to serious complications such as bleeding, perforation of the gastrointestinal wall or blockage of your large upper intestine.

So don't wait for the nasty later symptoms to occur. Go see the doctor now. Be sure of what you have. And then use these natural aids, along with his/her recommendations, to cure yourself . . . fast.

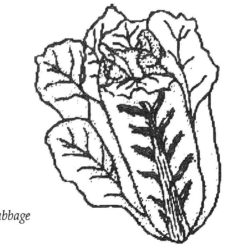

Cabbage

Summary

Remedies

- alfalfa
- ashwagandha
- cabbage and cabbage juice
- cowpeas
- crabmeat
- dark turkey meat
- eat regular meals of moderate size - don't overeat!
- lamb
- lean beef or pork
- licorice root
- nori
- oysters
- pepto-bismol and antacids (without aluminum)
- unripe, green plantains

Beneficial Supplements

- EPA's
- vitamin A
- vitamin B^6
- vitamin E
- zinc sulfate

Physical Remedies

- deep breathing exercises
- exercise
- meditation
- relaxation techniques

Caution! Avoid!

- abrasive roughage (nuts, popcorn, seeds)
- foods, fats and spices that make your stomach burn
- stress — don't let it get to you!
- too much alcohol
- too much caffeine

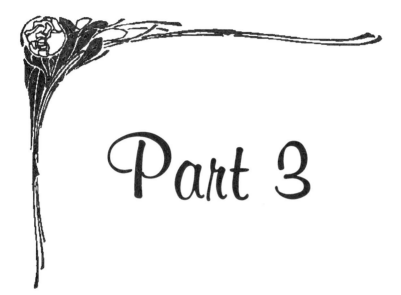

Part 3

19

Nutrition: The Key
To Second Youth

From the beginning of life, food has been a daily gratification. What a blessing, since it is absolutely essential to our existence. But, you must respect it if you want to stay healthy and young.

I have always loved food — any kind of food. How wonderful to put a tasty morsel in my mouth and savor the flavor and texture. My senses of smell and touch, together with my taste buds, find such a delight in it. Many emotions are satisfied by the process and I am in awe of the magnificence of it.

Imagine the tremendous range of benefits that food consumption produces. It soothes the savage beast in you when you are angry . . . placates your frustrations . . . rewards you in your triumphs . . . enhances your social get-togethers . . . consoles you in your grief, defeat and troubles . . . and, most important, fuels your body with energy and the elements to keep your body functions in action.

Are you one of those people who loves to eat and can't seem to control your weight? Or are you the size you want to be, but feel sluggish and old because your energy level won't let you keep up with the younger generation?

Unfortunately, the value of good eating habits is not considered until you have a problem with your body. From the time you were a baby, you probably never thought of any food being detrimental to your health and well-being. Everyone knows that sweets are delectable, spicy foods are so tasty, salt enhances almost all foods, and fats (butter, oils, meat fat) add flavor to our meals.

You grow up lasciviously enjoying "junk" foods and sweets because they taste so good and everyone is doing it. They are even given as rewards and tokens of love because they are so enjoyable. No one ever told you that these tasty morsels might shorten your longevity.

But, you can almost equate these foods with drugs. They feel so good and are so dangerous when abused.

"How can food be dangerous for you?" I can hear you saying, "and how much of a so-called dangerous food category constitutes a danger level anyway?"

The sad fact is that each individual's body chemistry reacts differently from someone else's so it is impossible to say definitely that 50 lbs. of meat fat over a period of one year will clog your arteries and cause a stroke or heart attack. Or that 50 lbs. of salt sprinkled on your food over a period of a year will cause your blood pressure to reach a dangerous level. For some, it will!

How do you know if you fall into that category? Are you willing to risk reaching the point of no return in order to find out?

Here are only some of the possible results of not monitoring your intake of the detrimental food categories.

Alcohol

Deterioration of the brain cells, loss of memory, obesity, kidney failure, sclerosis of the liver, stomach ulcers, intestinal ulcers, death.

Fats

Clogged arteries, high cholesterol, strokes, heart attacks, obesity, breathing problems, digestive tract problems, gall bladder attacks, gout, arthritis, foot and joint problems, sluggishness, and ultimately . . . death.

Sugar

Hypertension, hypotension, diabetic coma, tooth decay, obesity, imbalance in body chemistry, death.

Salt

Water retention, heart attacks, clogged arteries, headaches, kidney failure, death.

Spices

Certain physical conditions cannot tolerate the hot spices ... stomach ulcers, ulcerative colitis, cancer, gall bladder, death.

What a shame we don't have mandatory in-depth education at an early age, or for parents who are responsible for the eating habits of their children. It is so easy to learn something the right way from the beginning and so hard, almost impossible, to break habits that have been florishing for 20 or more years. It's like trying to reprogram your whole way of life which, in many instances, is exactly what has to be done in order to save your life or make it better.

When you were young, your healthy body rebounded so easily when you naively abused it by wantonly satisfying your gustatory desires. As you grow older, however, your body becomes weary of its battle to correct the effects of that abuse and starts to break down.

Well, your Second Youth is in your control and all you have to do is adopt a healthy eating pattern.

"Oh, it's easy for you to say. I've been trying all my life to eat the right foods," you say. "First, one diet, then another, but I seem to be fighting a losing battle." Familiar words, spoken by the majority of people.

Don't despair — there is hope. This miraculous organism is reparable and many illnesses and aging processses have been reversed through the proper use of food. Throughout this book, you will find my conclusions, after years of research and experimentation, which have given me the healthy, vital, strong and youthful body that brings so much pleasure to my lifestyle.

There are so many food categories that are healthy, energy-producing, helpful to our outer appearance, healing and, believe it or not, very tasty! Once you reprogram your taste buds to appreciate the natural flavors of food, you will find it most enjoyable to eat sensibly and healthfully. When you start feeling renewed energy and zest for life, see a strong healthy body taking shape, realize the alertness of a clear mind, and regain your sexual vigor, you will thank yourself for taking charge of your fate.

Let's look at foods that will be your helpers on the road to living longer and staying younger.

- beans
- fish
- fruits
- grains
- legumes
- occasional lean red meats

- plenty of water and natural, unsweetened fruit juices
- spices, herbs and lemon to add flavor
- vegetables
- white meats

Now, that gives you a very wide range of foods to eat that will enhance your life and bring on your Second Youth.

Enjoy!

20

Second Youth Slimness

$\mathcal{E}$veryone can lose weight permanently. Without sags in your body or lines in your face. Without torturous diets, or giving up the foods you love. Without even, in all cases, really dieting at all.

These are the newest findings of the obesity experts. And, by "obesity experts," I mean the doctors who specialize in losses of 20 pounds or more.

Over 90 percent of all women who suffer through an ordinary diet regain every ounce they have lost . . . and then more. But this is because they are using yesterday's knowledge, not the thrilling new facts that we've discovered today.

The world perceives you to be the image you present visually. If you fit the social image of the society in which you live, you will have a headstart on achieving a successful, happy life. It's cruel and unjust to be judged by your outward appearance, but that is a fact of life.

Let me give you some examples: American culture has set the image of a thin, well-shaped figure as the ideal. If you don't fit into that category, if instead you are obese ... hips out of proportion to your bust ... "love-handles" on your thighs ... "spare tire" at your waist ... etc., then you are perceived by others as a misfit, a loser, or out-of-control.

Or, perhaps, it leads you to believe that you are not as good as the other person. This creates a self-image that hinders the full expression of your existence. Because of your poor self-image, you perpetuate the belief that you are not good enough and life becomes a vicious cycle of insecurity and failures, of constantly trying to get it right, which saps your vitality and happiness.

Even worse, obesity takes a toll on your life by overstressing and causing breakdowns in the function of your body. An unhealthy body is an unhappy body, even a life-threatening one.

Diet or die!

❖ PERSONAL NOTE: At one time my scale read 192 lbs! That's 42 lbs. more than I weighed when I was 9 months pregnant with my son. I couldn't believe what was happening to me. I didn't want to believe I was *fat*.

I had always been proud that I had a figure that clients paid to photograph clothes on because my 120 lb. figure made their clothes look so good.

During this overweight period coinciding with my absence from modeling to have my children, and then to be a full-time homemaker, I made excuses for not buying new clothes. Each shopping expedition ended in depression when nothing made me look attractive. Why? Because, instead of remaining a size 8 or 9, I was trying on 12's and 14's. Finally, when I started struggling with the zippers of size 16's and the seams were straining, I realized I could no longer hide from reality. My figure was beginning to spread like molten lava and, if it wasn't checked, I was on my way to obesity and all the dangers that go along with that.

I felt sluggish and, although I loved dancing and sports, my excuse for not participating was that I was now a lady approaching middle age. The truth was that I didn't have the energy to move my growing body and I felt really self-conscious about my middle-aged spread.

How was I going to stop my craving for food when I loved the taste of it all? Eating seemed to be my most enjoyable exercise. It was very satisfying. You name it — I savored it;

there was no food my taste buds would turn down. And, to add to the folly, I really thought I was controlling my intake.

When I did start dieting, I realized I had not only been eating my own meal, but I was also finishing all the leftovers. In the process of cooking for my family and friends, I probably ate as much as I served them, thinking I was only "tasting." Then, between meals and while watching TV in the evening, I found myself "munching." Eating made me feel good. It gave me a sense of fulfillment.

I had another factor to contend with. My dearest friend! We were models who worked together for many years. Her slender figure made me feel more self-conscious so I would eat more to satisfy my frustration. I had to really pull myself together and turn my frustration into *determination*. "If she can do it, so can I!" became my motto, my silent chant.

First, I had to overcome using food as my psychological crutch and take control of my body. I decided to try different diet and exercise programs. My body needed a complete reversal of its "full-steam-ahead" eating syndrome.

When nothing worked, I gave up the fight. I was defeated, until . . .

To sum up my dieting experience, I yo-yoed up and down until I was finally tipping the scale at a hefty 180 pounds (60 lbs. more than I should have weighed). Yes, at age 45 I was not just overweight, I was obese. I was not just unhappy about the way I looked, I was scared out of my wits. My blood pressure, which had always been like a teenager's, shot up with my weight. My husband, who was only a few years older than me, died from an overworked heart due to *his* overweight. I had nightmares that I would be next.

I went to see dieting doctors and general health doctors, all of whom warned me that I would be deathly sick unless I lost weight and none of whom could help me keep it off for more than a month or two.

So, when their methods did not work, I developed my own plan. ❖

The yo-yo cycle *can* be broken. I did it, even before this new information was in. And since the days when I fought fat and won, new discoveries — thrilling new discoveries — have been made about food cures for overweight, especially through herbs and spices.

I wish I had known these secrets then so I wouldn't have had to spend so much of my time in a struggle that, for you, may now be almost effortless. I give you the results of my research.

My Method For Healthy Weight Control

Firm and Flaunt Your Fat

I had to go back to work and the only way I knew to make good money was by modeling. So, as my first step, I embarked on a serious exercise and toning program. Even though my weight did not drop off, my body began to take on a firm and shapely form. I no longer felt that I had to hide my fat. I was a larger version of what I used to be when I was 120 lbs.

This worked well enough for me to make a comeback as a full-figured model.

Yes, at first it was mortifying to present myself in my over-weight state to professionals who remembered me when I weighed 120. But they judged me to be highly presentable to the American public and put me to work as a representative of what a larger-sized woman could look like. The fact that they actually paid me for my extra pounds gave a much needed boost to my self-esteem.

What is the lesson for you? Simply this. You probably do not have to make a living on your looks, but the world still judges you by them. You can firm and shape those pounds at exactly the same time that you begin to lose them. Your first step towards losing weight is to follow the easy stretches and exercises I give you in this book. Soon you will be able to put your best foot forward and carry yourself with pride.

If you combine these simple exercises with the food rules I'm about to give you, the results will be striking. In weeks, friends will say, "How many inches did you lose from your waist?" Your visual weight loss will be many times your actual weight loss.

Don't be discouraged if the scale still registers the same weight. Muscles gain weight as they become stronger. The fat and flab will disappear and the weight will be distributed to the proper places. That is why you will appear to have lost weight. I find it more realistic and encouraging to judge my progress by taking my measurements instead of jumping on a scale every day.

You get an immediate reward, because you look 100% better. Plus you will get a long term permanent benefit because your body will actually be in a healthier state.

Besides, and equally as important, by doing these stretches and exercises from the very beginning, you strengthen your power of discipline and stick-to-itness. You regain control over the outline of your body. You regain confidence that you can remodel and reduce that body.

To lose weight permanently you must first feel good about yourself. And the easiest way I know to do this is to stretch and exercise your way back into control of your own figure.

When you are letting those stretches and exercises make the most of your full-fashioned figure, and you are reaping compliments, it is then far easier to undertake a sensible, easy, well-balanced reducing program. You are no longer as frantic to have quick results. And, above all, you are nowhere near as discouraged when — after the first drop in weight — you seem to plateau for a few days.

To lose weight permanently you must first feel good about yourself.

Eat Your Way to Healthy Living

Since you are now becoming firmer every day, and your outline is shrinking daily, you can afford to accept the only way to lose pounds permanently — slow and steady. Remember, throughout this entire regimen, your friends and family will think that you are losing many more pounds than you really are. Your sense of desperation, of crises, of rush-rush-rush will no longer be necessary.

Because of this, you will not need to deprive yourself or your taste buds. You will not trigger your body into slowing down its fat-burning powers because it thinks you have suddenly been placed in a state of famine. You will not be overcome by fatigue, or constant irritation, or uncontrollable binges.

Now that you have your stretching and exercising in place, you are going to place your food intake in control as well. How are you going to do this? This easily —

What makes you fat is fat!

If you eat fat, you will become fat.

What makes you fat is fat!

If you eat fat, you will become fat. Fat from outside your body makes fat on the inside of your body.

Fat can kill you!

Body fat, the fat that clogs every pore of your system, causes many complications and negative reactions in your system. Your body has a difficult time digesting fat so you get a reaction, as though the body were saying, "Hey! If you don't take care of me properly, you're going to suffer." And, oh, how you suffer for your lack of discipline!

If you don't eat fat, you will burn up the fat that's already in your body.

So what do you do about it? Simple. You just cut down on that deadly fat consumption.

How do you cut down on that deadly fat? Mathematically. Even if you never passed grade-school arithmetic, you can easily regulate your diet and lose weight permanently.

Limit your total fat intake to less than 30% of your daily calories. Limit your saturated fat intake to less than 10% of your daily calories.

On the new Nutrition Facts food label, saturated fat is a part of the total fat listed. It is listed separately because saturated fat is the most deadly fat. The Dietary Guidelines, prepared by the US Department of Agriculture, recommend limiting saturated fat to less than 10 percent of calories, or about one-third of total fat intake.

This is where the mathematics come in. And very simple mathematics it is. Here is the formula to follow:

Each gram of fat is 9 calories.

9 x fat grams per serving = X (fat calories per serving).

X divided by the number of calories = % of fat per serving.

On the following page is a reproduction of the new food label with information on how to read it. For more information there are pamphlets published as a public service by the US Food and Drug Administration and the US Department of Agriculture. (See addresses at the end of this chapter.) They have made it very easy for you to know the Nutrition Facts for every food you buy.

Example:

There are 12 grams of fat per serving on the package label. 9 x 12 = 108 fat calories. They can round out the number to 110.

The label says there are 250 calories per serving.

108 fat calories divided by 250 total calories = 43%. That product has a high fat content.

If you had one serving (one cup/8 oz.) of the above food, you would have had 108 fat calories or 12 grams. Two servings would give you 216 fat calories or 24 grams. It adds up fast, so be sure to keep track of your daily fat intake.

The New Food Label

- **The new heading** signals a new Nutrition Facts label.
- There are more consistent and realistic **serving sizes,** in both household and metric measures.
- The new term, **Calories from Fat,** helps consumers meet dietary guidelines that recommend people get no more than 30 percent of their calories from fat each day. Remember, it's your total consumption over the whole day, and not the percentage in one food or meal that's important.
- Use the **% Daily Values** to easily compare products and to quickly tell if a serving of a food is high or low in nutrients.
- The **Daily Values** that have been set for certain nutrients are listed on larger packages for both a 2,000- and a 2,500-calorie diet. (*See* Macaroni and Cheese label on next page.) This information is based on current dietary guidance and can help you understand the basics of a good diet and plan healthy meals.
- The **list of nutrients** covers those most important to the health of today's consumers, most of whom need to worry about getting too much of certain nutrients (fat, for example) rather than too few vitamins or minerals, as in the past.
- **Ingredients** still will be listed in descending order of weight. The list now will be required on almost all foods, even standardized ones such as mayonnaise and bread. The sources of some ingredients, such as certain flavorings, will be stated by name to help people better identify ingredients that they avoid for health, religious or other reasons.
- Claims may be made linking a nutrient or food to the risk of a chronic disease — but only if the nutritional makeup of the food meets certain conditions. (*See* Macaroni and Cheese label on next page.)

KEY: g = grams (about 28 grams = 1 ounce)
       mg = milligrams (1,000 milligrams = 1 gram)

You can believe the claims on the label because new guidelines ensure that nutrient claims mean the same on every product. Use this Macaroni and Cheese label as an example.

MACARONI AND CHEESE RICH IN CALCIUM
Net Wt 16 ¼ oz (456 g)
(See label for nutritional information)

Regular exercise and a healthy diet with enough calcium helps teen and young adult white and Asian women maintain good bone health and may reduce their risk of osteoporosis later in life.

INGREDIENTS: WATER, ENRICHED MACARONI (ENRICHED FLOUR [NIACIN,FERROUS SULFATE (IRON),THIAMINE MONONITRATE AND RIBOFLAVIN], EGG WHITE), FLOUR, CHEDDAR CHEESE (MILK, CHEESE CULTURE, SALT, ENZYME), SPICES, MARGARINE (PARTIALLY HYDROGENATED SOYBEAN OIL, WATER, SOY LECITHIN, MONO- AND DI-GLYCERIDES, BETA CAROTENE FOR COLOR, VITAMIN A PALMITATE), AND MALTODEXTRIN.

Nutrition Facts

Serving Size 1 cup (228g)
Servings Per Container 2

Amount Per Serving

Calories 250   Calories from Fat 110

	% Daily Value*
Total Fat 12g	**18%**
Saturated Fat 3g	**15%**
Cholesterol 30mg	**10%**
Sodium 470mg	**20%**
Total Carbohydrate 31g	**10%**
Dietary Fiber 0g	**0%**
Sugars 5g	
Protein 5g	

Vitamin A 4%	•	Vitamin C 2%
Calcium 20%	•	Iron 4%

*Percent Daily Values are based on a 2,000 calorie diet. Your daily values may be higher or lower depending on your calorie needs:

	Calories:	2,000	2,500
Total Fat	Less than	65g	80g
Sat Fat	Less than	20g	25g
Cholesterol	Less than	300mg	300mg
Sodium	Less than	2,400mg	2,400mg
Total Carbohydrate		300g	375g
Dietary Fiber		25g	30g

Calories per gram:
Fat 9   •   Carbohydrate 4   •   Protein 4

• **Calories per gram** shows the calorie content of the energy-producing nutrients.

❖ Here is a guideline of daily totals to follow

Calories	Total Fat – 30%	Total Saturated Fat – 10%
1600	480 cal./53 gr. or less	160 cal./18 gr. or less
2000	600 cal./66 gr. or less	200 cal./22 gr. or less
2500	750 cal./83 gr. or less	250 cal./28 gr. or less

You can figure the number of grams of fat that provide 30% of calories in your daily diet as follows:

A. Multiply your total day's calories by 0.30 to get your calories from fat per day.

Example: 2,200 calories x 0.30 = 660 calories from fat.

B. Divide calories from fat per day by 9 (each gram of fat has 9 calories) to get grams of fat per day.

Example: 660 calories from fat ÷ 9 = 73 grams of fat.

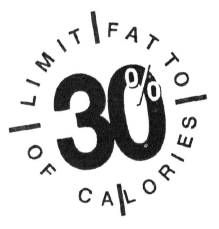

Daily Servings

- *Fats, Oils & Sweets:* use sparingly
- *Milk, Yogurt & Cheese Group:* 2–3 servings
- *Meat, Poultry, Fish, Dry Beans, Eggs & Nuts Group:* 2–3 servings
- *Vegetable Group:* 3–5 servings
- *Fruit Group:* 2–4 Servings
- *Bread, Cereal, Rice & Pasta Group:* 6–11 servings

On the opposite page is a reproduction of The Food Guide Pyramid published as a public service by the U.S. Department of Agriculture. See address at the end of this chapter.

Looking at the Pieces of the Pyramid

The Food Guide Pyramid emphasizes foods from the five major food groups shown in the three lower sections of the Pyramid. Each of these food groups provides some, but not all, of the nutrients you need. Foods in one group can't replace those in another. No one food group is more important than another — for good health, you need them all.

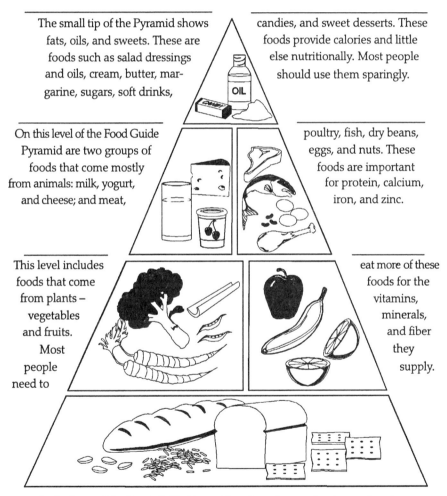

The small tip of the Pyramid shows fats, oils, and sweets. These are foods such as salad dressings and oils, cream, butter, margarine, sugars, soft drinks, candies, and sweet desserts. These foods provide calories and little else nutritionally. Most people should use them sparingly.

On this level of the Food Guide Pyramid are two groups of foods that come mostly from animals: milk, yogurt, and cheese; and meat, poultry, fish, dry beans, eggs, and nuts. These foods are important for protein, calcium, iron, and zinc.

This level includes foods that come from plants – vegetables and fruits. Most people need to eat more of these foods for the vitamins, minerals, and fiber they supply.

At the base of the Food Guide Pyramid are breads, cereals, rice, and pasta — all foods from grains. You need the *most* servings of these foods each day.

Any healthy diet must include foods from all of the five major food groups. The Pyramid shows you the proportions of each group that make up a healthy diet.

At the top of the Pyramid is the category most of you enjoy eating. But beware! A little is a lot. Use sparingly, because these foods will put you at high risk for disease and ill health.

Simple Rules To Follow To Remain Permanently Healthy and Slim

1. Have red meat once a week. No more. And trim all visible fat off it.

2. Have as much fowl as you want. Chicken, turkey, quail, etc. But, before you cook it, pull off its skin. That skin is almost pure fat. Don't even give it to the dog; just throw it in the garbage.

3. Eat all kinds of fish as often as possible. This includes such "fatty fish" as salmon, mackerel, sardines, etc. You can eat the fat because it's the kind of fat that burns off your body fat. The Omega-3 fatty acids found in fish are beneficial in counteracting all the maladies that are brought on by those undigestable fats.

Without question you need lots of fowl and fish — you need them for energy in your body, and youthfulness, and a glow in your face.

4. You've got to eat every time you're hungry. Eat as many fruits, vegetables, and grain foods as you want. Any time. All the time. Stuff them in. Gorge yourself. Fill your stomach up until it feels like it's bursting. Have as much natural bread (without the additives) as you wish all day. Eat, eat. Have three full meals a day, plus three or more snacks a day, plus a little something before you go to bed. The trick here is to fill yourself up with the foods that won't make you fat and that will make you slim forever.

5. Have sugar if you want — as long as it's fruit sugar or honey. Regain again the knowledge that fruit sugar and honey are far sweeter than the condensed sugar you've been getting from processed foods. They are also incredibly healthier than that white killer.

6. If you must eat processed foods every so often, eat those with a minimum of fat. Read labels. Buy no processed food unless it lists its ingredients and Nutrition Facts on the label.

7. Ordinary chocolate is a no-no. But there are defanged chocolates that you can still have. These are tootsie rolls, low fat hot fudge, chocolate flavored syrup and chocolate flavored cereal. Carob has been used as a substitute for chocolate. It comes from an evergreen tree in the Mediterranean region that has edible pods (also called St. John's bread). Experiment with them. You'll be surprised how delicious, and appetizing, and satisfying they do become.

8. Beware of hydrogenated, unsaturated, undigestible oils, such as: coconut, palm, palm kernel and mineral oil. Saturated fat is also found in meats and dairy products.

9. Use only monosaturated fats, such as: olive oil, peanut oil and canola oil. Or polyunsaturated fats, such as: soybean oil, sunflower oil, corn oil, cottonseed oil and safflower oil for your salad dressings. These are health builders, not health destroyers.

10. If you drink alcohol, drink only one or two glasses a day — preferably before or during eating.

11. Keep your salt/sodium intake to a minimum. Sodium is found in carbonated beverages and bicarbonates, cured meats, lunch meats, most canned foods, dairy products (particularly processed cheese), packaged foods, condiments and sauces. Watch out for soy sauce — it has a high salt content. Salt/sodium can put you at risk for high blood pressure. If you already have high blood pressure, eliminate all salt/sodium from your diet.

If you follow these few simple rules, you will be on the right road to a healthier life. If, for example, you eat only complex carbohydrates, you just can't eat enough of them to gain weight. And if you don't supplement them with fat-laden foods, you just can't stuff enough of them down your mouth to keep you from losing weight, slowly and permanently.

Whether you weigh your food, or measure the portions you are going to serve yourself, remember you are not in prison, you're in life. Enjoy it. De-mechanize it. Don't be a diet machine. If you diligently follow the simple rules of a healthy diet, you will have fun losing weight. It's the only way it will stay off your body permanently.

Vary Your Meals with the Hundreds of Foods You Now Can Eat

Remember, you are finished with fad dieting forever. Since you are, decide every day for yourself which foods you want most that day. Be sure to choose from each of the five food categories. Follow your whims, your moods, and the best fruits and vegetables, etc. that are in season that day.

Follow your old favorites, innovate with new surprises. (I never thought I would like beans, for example, but now I find them delicious. And *Beano* takes their sting away.)

Also, once I memorized the rules above, I no longer had any qualms about an occasional indulgence in rich dishes, in fat dishes, or in junk food. But occasional is the key word here. It means, mathematically, only once every two weeks. The odd splurge does not make that much difference as long as your basic rules are maintained. This way, there is no guilt. Just make the following day a salad day, or a no protein day, or even a juice day that purifies your whole system.

Maintain a Regular Eating Schedule

According to Dr. C. Wayne Callaway of George Washington University of Medicine and Health Sciences, the three most common ways to cause weight gaining problems are starving, skipping and stuffing. Adopting a regular eating schedule is a crucial first step toward regulating your appetite. This means a well-balanced breakfast as well as lunch and dinner.

Have your meals at about the same time every day. However, you can vary the time of the four snacks every day that you should allow yourself.

This seven meal a day principle is called, as you probably already know, *grazing*. It works on the principle of eat, eat, eat. When you feel hungry, satisfy it. Only satisfy it according to the rules above.

Adopting a regular eating schedule is a crucial first step toward regulating your appetite.

As for breakfast, you must have it. This is absolutely essential. It fortifies you for the entire day. It energizes you for that entire day. It prevents mid-morning binges, and — believe it or not — mid-afternoon downers. Have, at the very minimum, rye, wheat or whole grain toast every morning.

Be Realistic ... Aim for Your Natural Body Weight

The essential point is to stay young and healthy, not to conform to some arbitrary thinness fashion. You are out to lose the bad pounds, the ones that overburden your heart, your back, that aggravate adult onset diabetes or make you short of breath. In other words, the excess baggage that shortens your life.

Unless you are born to be lean, unless slimness is in your genes, you are wasting your time by over-dieting. You were meant to be a certain natural body weight. If you follow this plan for any reasonable time, you will arrive at that natural body weight for you. You will know this when your scale no longer goes down, or goes up, but stays at the same level for a few months. There, you are at the weight nature intended you to be. You will look your best at that weight, no more and no less. Both your body and your face will be at their most attractive there. Reach it, hold it, enjoy it.

Age is also a factor. Most women gain between 10 or 15 pounds around or just after middle age. Look around you, notice that most men do the same thing. But they have a huge advantage over us: it doesn't seem to bother them nearly as much.

And it shouldn't bother you. You want to look attractive, not thin.

According to Dr. Janet Polivy, a psychologist at the University of Toronto, "It's time we started treating body weight more like height, as a biologically determined trait."

However, if you try to go beyond your natural, determined weight, you will put too much strain on your mind and body, and you will begin yo-yoing again. I prefer to keep my flesh firm by continuing to exercise, rather than by having less of it. I prefer to insure the renewed youth and energy that satisfactory and intelligent eating has given me.

At 5'7", and 150 pounds, I like the way I look. So do men (I have no problem at all finding those who propose marriage by the second or third date). My agents and my casting directors must like the way I look, too (I have no problems finding work). I am, in short, living proof that you can be built for comfort, and still be glamorous. So why be taken in by the "thinness industry?" As you must know by now, in real life people are tired of the "anorexic look," of women so skinny that you can sense the vultures circling overhead. Be your buoyant, well-endowed, healthy self and enjoy it!

Use Water To Wash Weight Away

What we often think is hunger, may actually be only thirst. Especially as we grow older, the two sensations merge and become confused. That's why you should always test what you really want: food or water.

The method is simple. If you have the urge for a fat-filled snack, say chocolate ice-cream, sip a glass of iced water instead. The cold is there. The liquid is there. After a few moments, you may find yourself completely satisfied, and you haven't taken in a single calorie.

In the same way, before you sit down to every meal, have a plain-water cocktail first. That's a full glass of water, no less. Or, at night, put a touch of wine in it. Or, if you wish, make it a weak wine spritzer. Get your liquid first, and your body will want less fat.

After you've had your water cocktail, wait five minutes, if possible, before you begin the meal. Especially if you're drinking iced water, do not take too much of it with the meal itself. It bloats you, and weakens your digestive powers.

If possible, and you can make it completely possible, sip water all day long. Try to take six 8 oz. glasses a day. This will have two effects on your body: first, it will act as a natural diuretic, and second it will flush the internal fat out of your body. You'll use water to wash your excess weight away.

You'll never take another diuretic drug, with their dangerous side effects and the ever-present danger of addiction, when all you need to do is turn on the tap.

Try to skip all the sodas, diet or not, since they're either filled with sugars or unnatural chemicals. Our internal body is mostly made of water. You have a little pure lake of water inside your cells. Like any other lake, it must have fresh, clean rivers running in and out of it to keep it pure.

One of my favorite purifiers is fresh water with the juice of a lemon squeezed into it. I even put the rest of the lemon in it and keep it in the refrigerator to refresh myself throughout the day.

With my plan, which has been proven by dozens of my friends who are models, and dozens of my friends who are housewives, and dozens of my friends who are in business, the fat floats out of your body. Your cheeks will bloom again. The freshness and fullness of youth comes back into your face. And you weigh less and less and less.

Caffeine Burns Fat

The caffeine released by coffee, guarana, maté, cola and tea not only wakes you up, its energizing effect also promotes the burning of fat. One hundred milligrams of caffeine daily has been shown to increase your metabolic rate by about 10 percent. That means you've found a terribly satisfying and effective way to burn up an extra 100 or more calories a day. I have a hardy cup of coffee after breakfast, and a delicious cup of regular tea in the early afternoon. However, because too much caffeine is counter-effective and turns on the jitters, I have only herbal tea at night. I do not have cream or sugar in my coffee or tea. My only whole milk of the day goes into my morning coffee. Lemon is delightful in my regular tea and the herbal teas have a wonderful flavor all their own.

A note about caffeine: *some of you might have an adverse physical reaction to caffeine. If you do, please follow your doctor's advice.*

Plants That Promote Weight Loss

The evidence is now overwhelming that spicy food which burns your mouth burns up calories by increasing the rate of your body's metabolism. Any food does this slightly, of course, but according to a study by Oxford Polytechnic researchers, the hot stuff boosts it by 25 percent.

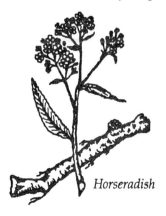

Horseradish

In other words, if part of your problem is a sluggish metabolism (and this applies to 99 percent of women over the age of 40), add a little spice to your life. Go primarily for the capsicum, as in cayenne pepper, chili pepper, Tabasco sauce, etc., but curry, fresh ginger, horseradish and hot mustard can rev up your system as well.

Other energizing botanicals include damiana, ephedra, ginseng and schisandra, all available at herbalists or health food stores. They are marvelous aids for weight control because they make you want to get up and go, rather than slouch on the couch. Siberian ginseng always gives me a lift, for example, and sometimes that is all I need to stop from pigging out when I feel blue.

If you have a sluggish thyroid, or suspect that you do, try kelp from your health food store. This normalizes the gland's activities without having to rely on drugs.

Chlorella detoxifies your system, helping your body rid itself of accumulated fatty waste.

And, of course, there are the fiber-rich foods. They are super nutritious and they also make you feel full. Very full. They include whole grains and other starchy foods, ranging from such familiar staples as barley, bran, oats, pasta, rye and whole wheat bread to such less readily available varieties as glucomannan, long used by the Japanese, or spirulina, a classic African source, and wheatgrass.

Utensils That Help You Lose Weight

Weight control is often more a question of simple, smart moves than drastic measures. And some involve the utensils you use to prepare food, not just the food itself.

For example, a blender allows you to purée vegetables to use as thickeners for cream soups and sauces instead of a roux. Add a dollop of cream at the end, if you want.

A clay cooker allows meats to simmer slowly in their own juices without having to lard or baste them with fat.

Non-stick, teflon pans allow you to sauté food, using far less oil or butter, but still keeping the full flavor. Slice, chop and quick stir-fry in a wok or cast-iron pan for the same purpose.

A double-boiler allows you to warm up leftovers without adding butter or oil. If you do not have one, you can always improvise by placing the food you want to warm up in a small pot, either over or in a larger one that contains boiling or simmering water.

A steamer retains the flavor as well as the vitamins in vegetables (as you know, overcooking vegetables takes everything out of them). Otherwise, just cook them quickly in boiling water, lift out and drain (do not use a lid when cooking greens or they will turn an unappetizing gray).

Or, quickly sauté them in butter and garlic or a vinaigrette dressing. Then all you need is a sprinkling of herbs and a squirt of lemon juice to bring out the flavor.

Supplements That Put Your Appetite To Sleep

You probably have heard about taking amino acid concentrates to curb your appetite. Unlike diet pills, which I do not recommend at all, they are considered to be food supplements. As such, they are readily available at health food stores and many pharmacies.

L-glutamine, which the body produces in small amounts by itself, quiets your craving for sweets. In combination with L-phenylalanine, it releases a brain hormone that tells your brain when you have had enough to eat.

Any good source of protein — beef, in particular — contains L-phenylalanine, but it must be taken in pure form as a supplement to be really psychoactive, according to Dr. William H. Lee, R.Ph., Ph.D. He adds that, to be effective, these supplements also need an intake of vitamin C and B^6. Furthermore, they should not be taken if you suffer from high blood pressure, the genetic disease phenylketonuria (PKU), or if your doctor has prescribed a monoamine oxidase (MAO) inhibitor.

Other fat-burning supplements include L-carnitine, Q-10 (CoEnzyme Q-10), GO (Gamma-Oryzanol) and DHEA. I have seen much documentation on the efficiency of all four. They certainly give your waste-burning powers a boost. I have used them, with amazing effects.

They're all sold in health food stores, but if you have any questions, consult a nutritionally-trained physician. Or a recommended nutrition specialist.

❖ PERSONAL NOTE:

When I was modeling as a size 8, I had to keep my weight at 120 lbs. My doctor prescribed diet pills. They worked for a while, but I found myself becoming addicted to them.

My personality was becoming manic-depressive. My moods would swing from very happy-go-lucky to depression and fear of being with people. It took more and more dosage to maintain what I felt was necessary to stay thin and keep my energy level up. My sense of values changed. My common sense went into hiding.

When I realized what was happening, I asked the doctor to help me withdraw from my addiction. It wasn't easy!

Since then, I became determined to find a way to stay slim and sane without those chemicals. I did. And, I did lose the weight I needed to lose, without using diet pills, and I *kept* it off without them.

There will never be an end to "miracle" diet pills. They are sold to you in the press, on television, and even in some of the best doctor's offices. As I write this chapter, for example, I see 12 books, 24 advertisements and 36 doctors ready to turn me into a drug addict, and make a fortune.

Diet pills drug you. They turn you into a robot for a number of weeks. They do strange and disastrous things to your mind and body. They make you lose all those otherwise wonderful weeks of your life, which you will never, never gain back.

In the long run, you go back to the same weight or become even heavier than before. Even worse, you have picked up a yearning to have a pill do your life's work for you.

Diet pills are a substitute, not for willpower, but for knowledge. Once you have the knowledge I have given you above, you'll lose more weight comfortably than you could with any diet pill in the world.

If you depend on pills for diet, won't you then begin to depend on pills for sex, for serenity, for standing up for yourself, and for every other task that life presents to you . . .

Of course, I would like to take a pill and see my excess fat disappear. And, of course I would like to take a pill every month after, and never see an ounce of it reappear.

But no, nature does not work that way. Probably for a very good reason: nature wants you strong and independent, so you can control your own body. And, so you can shape your Second Youth for the long and beautiful rest of your life.

No one — especially you — should embark on diet pills casually. Their validity is unproven. Consult a physician first for your personal nutrition plan, or use the far easier plan given you above.

As always, nature is the cure. Learn to work with her and your overweight will become a memory. Your Second Youth will be an expression of your new lease on life.

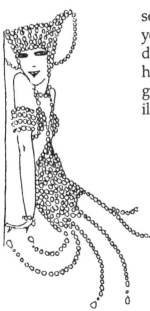

P.S. There is also an answer to presenting an image of perfection, even if your body isn't. That is in the way you dress, apply makeup, and care for your hair. In my chapter on Imaging, I will give you different ways to create the illusion of a perfect body.

As for the physical conditioning of your body, my chapters on Exercise and Face Exercises, will give you additional information on how to actually create the perfect body.

Good Luck! Stick with my program and I guarantee that you will bring more vitality and happiness into your life!

SUMMARY

Ways To Fight Obesity

- Accept that: "slow and steady" is the safest way to lose weight.
- Maintain a diet low in fat, saturated fat, and salt.
- Accept your nature-intended body weight and maintain it.
- Learn how to create the illusion of a well-balanced figure with the way you dress, apply makeup and style your hair.
- Reshape and firm your body through:

  - ❖ aerobic machines (treadmill, stairmaster rowing)
  - ❖ dancing
  - ❖ exercise
  - ❖ massage
  - ❖ swimming
  - ❖ walking
  - ❖ yoga

Spices, Plants and Supplements That Promote Weight Loss

Spices Such As:

- cayenne pepper
- chili pepper
- curry
- fresh ginger
- horseradish
- hot mustard
- tabasco sauce

Plants Such As:

- chlorella
- damiana
- ephedra
- ginseng
- kelp
- schisandra
- spirulina
- wheatgrass

Overall Nutritional Principles

- EAT
  - beans and legumes
  - fish
  - fruit
  - grains
  - lean meat
  - pasta (without butter and sauces)
  - skinless fowl and poultry
  - vegetables

- DRINK
  - fruit juices
  - water

Drink at least 48 ounces of water a day!

- AND REMEMBER

  - Cut your total fat intake to 30% or less of your calories and your saturated fat intake to 10% or less of your daily calories.
  - Eat three well-balanced, moderate meals a day.
  - Have nutritional snacks between meals to curb your appetite.
  - Use only olive, canola, peanut, soybean, safflower, sunflower, corn, and cottonseed oils.

Supplements Such As:
(*Note Contraindications Mentioned in Chapter*)

- amino acids
- DHEA
- GO
- L-carnitine
- L-glutamine
- L-phenylalanine
- Q-10
- vitamin B^6
- vitamin C

Do not use diet pills unless under your doctor's supervision!

Use In Moderation Or Eliminate

- bicarbonates
- canned foods
- carbonated beverages
- condiments and sauces (particularly soy sauce}
- cured meats
- dairy products
- lunch meats
- packaged foods
- salt (eliminate), use lemon juice and herbs for seasoning instead
- white sugar (eliminate), use fruit sugar (fructose) and honey
- AND REMEMBER:
    - drink no more than 2 cups of a caffeine beverage a day
    - drink no more than 2 glasses of an alcoholic beverage a day

Food Preparation Utensils That Help You Lose Weight

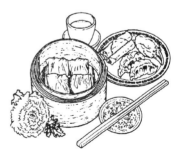

- blenders to purée vegetables for sauces and soups
- utensils for cooking without oil:
    - a wok
    - clay crock pots
    - double-boilers
    - non-stick coated pans
    - steamers

There are many free pamphlets available from the places listed below which give you a whole realm of information on Dietary Guidelines and the new Nutrition Facts food label.

The United States Department of Agriculture
6505 Belcrest Road, Hyattsville, MD 20782.
The Food Safety Hotline is (toll free) 1-800-535-4555.

Food and Drug Administration
Department of Health and Human Services
5600 Fishers Lane (HFE-88), Rockville, MD 20857.

Look in the Blue Pages of your telephone book for the local office.

The Seafood Hotline is (toll free) 1-800-FDA-4010

The American Heart Association, National Center, 7272 Greenville Ave., Dallas, TX 75231
(toll free) 1-800-242-8721

Catalogs that list many helpful booklets for free or at a small fee can be requested from:

Consumer Information Catalog
S. James, Consumer Information Center
4D, P.O.Box 100. Pueblo, CO 81002

Office of Publications
U.S. General Services Administration,
Washington, D.C. 20405

21

My Daily Vitamins and Minerals

ere is a list of my daily vitamins and minerals!

- ❖ **Schiff:** Natural Super Calcium "1200" with vitamin D, 400 I.U. Source: calcium carbonate, vitamin D — fish liver oil in a natural base of vegetable oil and lecithin.

- ❖ **Schiff:** Natural "Time Release" Vitamin C, 1500 mg (twice a day). Source: vegetable, in a natural base of rose hips, vegetable oil and silica cellulose.

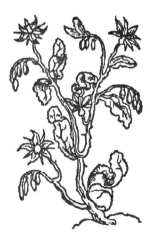

Borage

- ❖ **Schiff:** Natural Vitamin B^6, 100 mg. Source: pyridoxine HCI, in a natural base of whole brown rice concentrate including the hull, polishings and the kernel, terra alba, acacia, vegetable oil and food glaze.

257

❖ **Schiff**: Super B-Complex with B^{12}, including:

- vitamin B^1 (thiamine mononitrate) 30 mg
- vitamin B^2 (riboflavin) 35 mg
- vitamin B^6 (pyridoxine HCl) 15 mg
- niacinamide 50 mg
- vitamin B^{12} (cobalamin conc.) 100 mg
- biotin 0.3 mg
- pantothenic acid (d-cal pantothenate) 100 mg
- folic acid 0.4 mg
- choline bitartrate 50 mg
- Inositol 100 mcg
- Methionine 25 mcg
- PABA (p-aminobenzoic acid) 50 mg
- In a natural base of whole rice concentrate including the hull, polishings and the kernel, calcium sulfate, lecithin, silica, food glaze, vegetable oil and cellulose

❖ **Schiff:** Chelated Zinc, 50 mg. Source: zinc amino acid chelate/soy in a natural base of hydrolized vegetable protein, cellulose, vegetable oil, silica, dicalcium phosphate.

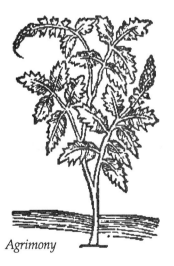

Agrimony

❖ **Schiff:** Natural Selene-E with Lecithin (Natural Antioxidants). Source: selenium (primary selenium yeast) 100 mcg, vitamin E (soy — 134.23 mg d-alpha tocopherol) 200 I.U., lecithin (soy beans) 640 mg. In a natural base of primary selenium yeast, lecithin, unesterified natural mixed tocopherols, soy bean oil, glycerine, vegetable oil and beeswax.

❖ **Duane Reade:** Natural Organic Vitamin E, 400 I.U. Source: d-alpha tocopheryl acetate and d-alpha tocopherol (from natural vegetable oils).

❖ **Duane Reade:** Therex M, including:

- vitamin A (palmitate) 5,500 I.U.
- vitamin C (ascorbic acid) 120 mg
- vitamin B^1 (thiamine mononitrate) 3 mg
- vitamin B^2 (riboflavin) 3.4 mg
- niacin (as niacinamide) 30 mg
- vitamin B^6 (as pyridoxine hydrochloride) 3 mg
- vitamin B^{12} (cyanocobalamin) 9 mcg
- vitamin D 400 I.U.
- vitamin E (as dl-tocopheryl acetate) 30 I.U.
- pantothenic acid (as calcium pantothenate) 10 mg
- folic acid 0.4 mg
- biotin 15 mcg

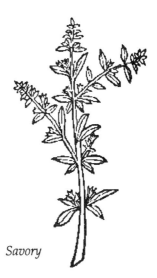

Savory

- calcium (as calcium carbonate) 40 mg
- iodine (as potassium iodide) 150 mcg
- iron (as ferrous fumarate) 27 mg
- magnesium (as magnesium oxide) 100 mg
- copper (as cupric sulfate) 2 mg
- zinc (as zinc sulfate) 15 mg
- manganese (as manganese sulfate) 5 mg
- chromium (from chromium yeast) 15 mcg

- selenium (from selenium yeast) 10 mcg
- molybdenum (from molybdenum yeast) 15 mcg
- potassium (as potassium chloride) 7.5 mg
- chloride (as potassium chloride) 7.5 mg

Vitamins and Minerals Daily Supplements

The following are incorporated into eight different capsules, and most of them are within one multi-vitamin/mineral capsule.

- vitamin A – 5,500 IU
- vitamin B^1 – 33 mg
- vitaminB^2 – 38 mg
- vitamin B^6 – 118 mg
- vitamin B^{12} – 109 mg
- vitamin C – 2120 mg
- vitamin D – 800 IU
- vitamin E – 1030 IU
- biotin – 18 mcg
- calcium (as calcium carbonate) – 1240 mg
- choline bitartrate – 50 mg
- chloride (as potassium chloride) – 7.5 mg
- chromium (from chromium yeast) – 15 mg
- copper (as cupric sulfate) – 2 mg
- folic acid – .8 mg
- inositol -100 mcg
- iodine (as potassium iodide) – 150 mcg
- iron (as ferrous fumarate) – 27 mg
- lecithin (from soy beans) – 640 mg
- magnesium (as magnesium oxide) – 100 mg
- manganese (as manganese sulfate) – 5 mg
- molybdenum (from molybdenum yeast) – 15 mcg
- methionine – 25 mg
- niacinamide – 80 mg
- paba (p-aminobenzoic acid) – 50 mg
- pantothenic acid (as calcium pantothenate) – 110 mg
- potassium (as potassium chloride) – 7.5 mg
- selenium (from selenium yeast) – 110 mg
- zinc (as zinc sulfate) – 15 mg
- zinc (zinc amino acid chelate/soy) – 50 mg

22

Physical Fitness: Stretching and Exercising Give New Life!

*W*elcome to the world of the beautiful, healthy and physically fit. By stretching and exercising, you will have taken the first step towards a more fulfilling life. Flexibility and the ability to move with strength and agility is the essence of a healthy, youthful body that defies the aging process.

Think of the complaints associated with aging, i.e.:

- ❖ "My back is killing me."
- ❖ "I can't keep up the pace I used to have when I was young."
- ❖ "My body feels like it's falling apart."
- ❖ "I haven't got the strength to keep going."
- ❖ "The old ticker isn't what it used to be."
- ❖ "I get so winded when I climb stairs or walk a distance."

Most people think of these as an inevitable part of life. They are, if you choose to live a sedentary lifestyle. But you can actually embrace a more fulfilling and enjoyable lifestyle by actively taking steps to strengthen and tone this miraculous body you live in.

261

Stretch and exercise your joints and bring elasticity back to your muscles.

You are as young as the flexibility your body gives you every day. Stretch and exercise that body, and you liberate its trapped energy.

Your joints age because they stiffen from lack of movement and lubrication. Stretch and exercise that body and you oil the joints and bring elasticity back to your muscles.

Your skin loses its tenacity and color because your circulation pump is not working as powerfully as it used to. Stretch and exercise your body and you will revive the power of your heart and arteries. The blood will flow more freely, bringing color and nutrition to the surface of your skin.

Why else are flexibility and strength important? They give you the ability to bend effortlessly. To stretch. To lift a child or grandchild from the ground without strain. To dance. To lean over your loved one and embrace him. To make love, and play long hours. And to forget that the word "stiffness" or "pain" ever existed.

Strong muscles will help lighten the load on your heart. And osteoporosis can be prevented by weight-bearing exercise, if started before the age of 40. Or, if weight-bearing exercise is started after the age of 50, osteoporosis can be slowed down and the bone loss can be halted. There are even studies now which show that weight-bearing exercise may help *stimulate* bone building.

When stretching and exercising, the emotional knots will be released from your muscles. The adrenalin that is generated will energize your mind and body, giving you a sense of well-being and an alertness to deal with stress in a more positive way.

The Second Youth body you are about to build is firm and strong. It is beautiful and desirable. And you can have it far more easily than you dreamed. The first step is the easiest exercise of all.

Getting Rid of the Myths That Are Blocking You From A Second Youth Body Today

Yes!! You *can* be fit — no matter what size you are — no matter what age you are — no matter what shape you're in right now!

Your body can be firm, beautiful, healthy and alive — no matter how much you weigh today — you don't *have* to be skinny.

No matter how much fatty tissue your body has, your muscles can be lengthened and strengthened so you can move easily and gracefully. A physically *fit* body is youthful and full of life, ready to take on whatever lies ahead.

Think about it for a moment. A firm 150 pounds looks far slimmer and far more youthful than 120 sagging, flabby pounds. Firm bodies have no pot bellies. No cellulite thighs. No hanging buttocks. No drooping breasts or floppy underarms.

As you progress in my firming program, you will find your weight being distributed to the right places so your body will be more properly proportioned. You may or may not lose weight because, even though you will burn some fat off, the muscles will weigh more as they develop. *Weight loss can only be achieved through a proper diet*, combined with exercise.

The purpose of exercise is to shape and firm the muscles so they can perform their best for you. Your body will look and feel better when you are in control of your muscles.

Trust me for two short weeks, and I'll prove — beyond a shadow of a doubt — that I can remove the figure problems that have plagued you for years.

I have my own ideas about *really effective* exercise. After all, my income depended on never allowing a figure problem of my own to show in the camera. Nor could I look tired or strained when I was in front of that camera. So the exercises I developed were easy, fast, and exhilarating instead of exhausting.

And above all, they were *emergency treatment* exercises. They did for my figure problems what a bandage does for a cut on your finger. They stopped the problems from getting worse *at once*, and they healed it so completely that — as long as you took care of it — it never came back.

You'll see the first results in two short weeks. I promise you this!

Looking Better Is Just the Beginning — Feeling Better Is Even More Important

When you stretch and exercise, you feel good. Your circulation improves. Your metabolism increases (helping you to lose weight). Your adrenalin starts flowing (generating more energy and positive thinking). Stiffness and tension are released. Aches and pains (produced by emotional stress and the lack of activity) drain right out of your body.

You will also find that, throughout the day, when tension and stress take over your body, a brief interlude of simple stretches will loosen you up and recharge your batteries. There is no need to limit yourself to a specific "exercise and stretch" time. Integrate it into your lifestyle whenever your body feels out of sync.

These stretches and exercises are designed so that anyone — even the elderly and handicapped — can do them. Many of them are performed on the floor. This puts less stress on your heart, vital organs and back. You can also do most of them while sitting in a chair.

If at all possible, I suggest the use of a trainer who is well educated in physical therapy. A good trainer can motivate you, monitor your progress, and make sure that you are doing the movements correctly.

It is important that you do stretches and exercises five days each week, without fail, in order to achieve your Second Youth goals.

In the beginning, you may experience sore muscles. This is only natural and is a sign that you are getting to muscles that haven't been used for a while. Those muscles are the ones that need toning the most.

A warm bath and gentle massage will relieve the soreness. As you strengthen your muscles, your body will respond by actually wanting to use those muscles more. And before you realize it, your body will be much more responsive and alive.

As you become more aware of your body and its muscular functions, you will be able to notice when your posture is working against you. For instance, allowing your abdominal muscles to hang out puts a tremendous strain on your back and can pull your vertebrae out of alignment or even cause a slipped disk. So, you'll learn the right way to " suck in your gut" and keep those abdominal muscles working.

No one thinks of slouched posture as pretty. Your chin doubles and triples — your shoulders drop and roll forward — your waist thickens and develops "spare tires." Who wants to look like that?!

Even worse than the outside appearance of a slovenly body is the harm that is happening inside to your muscles, organs, nerves and skeletal framework!

I *promise!* — if you incorporate just 15 minutes of stretching and exercising into your everyday lifestyle, you will strengthen and lengthen the muscles that control your posture.

When your body starts to firm up and take on a better shape, you will find a real pride in your presence. You will actually become more sexually appealing. Your sexuality will be liberated, no matter what your age. You will be further encouraged by the responses to the *new you!*

You will start to walk taller and carry your body with pride and grace. Good posture enhances your appearance. Your head is held proudly. Your shoulders look squared off. Your chest rises and allows your lungs to expand, bringing more air and oxygen into your body. Your tummy tucks in to support your back. Your buttocks tuck under, relieving the small of your back. Your waist becomes smaller because you have lifted your ribs off your hips. And you will start to lose your double chins!

What a pretty sight! Good posture tells the world how much you like yourself. It says, *"I am happy to be alive!"*

Remember! You are worth the small effort it takes to make your body healthy and attractive. You owe it to yourself to keep your machine in good working condition so make that promise to give yourself the best of life. *You won't regret it!*

You Have Only One Life And It's Up To You To Get The Most Enjoyment Out Of It!

Now, Let's Get Started —

My Simple Wake-up Routine:

> Note: This method of getting out of bed is particularly good for poor circulation. It also helps prevent pulled muscles and dislocated vertebrae.

When my eyes open or the alarm goes off, I lie there peacefully, allowing my senses to adjust to the new day.

I listen to the sounds of my world.

I breathe deeply and feel the surge of life flowing through my body.

❖ While lying there, I slowly stretch —

- First the right side (hand towards the top of the bed, foot towards the bottom of the bed) for a count of 5.

- Then the left side for a count of 5.

- Then both sides at the same time for a count of 5. (Picture a cat stretching upon awakening.)

❖ I pull my right knee up towards my chest and hold it with my hands for a count of 5 (relaxing and lengthening the muscles of my back).

- I release my knee and straighten my leg on the bed.

- Then I pull my left knee up towards my chest and hold it with my hands for a count of 5.

- I release my knee and straighten my leg on the bed.

❖ I rest my arms over my head and put the soles of my feet together, bending my legs in a froglike position. (If I am a little stiff, I cross my ankles and let my knees relax open. Then I bring my feet towards my buttocks, stopping where it feels comfortable.)

- I relax in this position for a count of 5, breathing deeply and letting a low sigh come out as an *"Ahh."*

- Then I straighten my legs and arms, and give them a full stretch once more to a count of 5.

❖ I rotate my feet in circles, first to the right for a count of 5 — then to the left for a count of 5. (This is good for the muscles and ligaments of the ankles.)

- Next, I flex my feet towards my head for a count of 5. And then point my feet down for a count of 5.

- Next, I curl my toes tightly for a count of 5. Then, I spread my toes wide for a count of 5.

❖ When I am ready to get up from my bed, I roll onto my side towards the edge of the bed.

- Placing both hands on the side towards the edge, I use them to push my upper body upright.

- At the same time, I swing my legs over the edge of the bed and come to a sitting position.

- I relax there for a minute as my body adjusts.

- Then I stand for another minute as my body adjusts to that stance.

Now I am ready to take on the day with vigor!

Neck Stretches

While I am taking my morning shower with the warm water loosening my neck muscles, I do my neck stretches. Neck muscles must be lengthened and strengthened. They support your head and the vertebrae in your neck. They give you the ability to move your head in all directions.

1. Raise your right arm towards the ceiling, then bend it over the top of your head and place your right hand over your left ear.

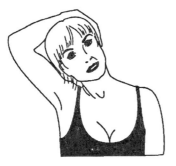

- Slowly let your head tilt to the right side (the weight of your arm will create a good stretch to the neck muscles).

- Relax into the stretch for a count of 5.
- Return your head to the upright position and lower your arm.
- Now raise your left arm towards the ceiling, then bend it over your head and place your left hand over your right ear.
- Slowly tilt your head to the left side.
- Relax into the stretch for a count of 5.
- Return your head to the upright position and lower your arm.

2. Raise your right arm and place your hand at the base of your skull behind your left ear.

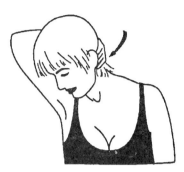

- Turn your face to a point halfway between the front and your right side.

- Slowly tilt your head down.
- Relax into the stretch for a count of 5.
- Lift your head, face forward and lower your arm.
- Raise your left arm and place your left hand on the base of your skull behind your right ear.
- Turn your face to a point between the front and your left side.
- Slowly tilt your head down.
- Relax into the stretch for a count of 5.
- Lift your head, face forward and lower your arm.

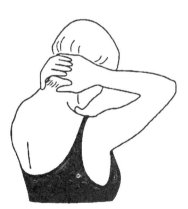

3. Raise both arms and place your hands at the base of your skull.

- Slowly tilt your head forward.
- Relax into the stretch for a count of 5.
- Lift your head and lower your arms.

Repeat the above stretches in sequence each day!

The PC Muscles

A group of muscles that are seldom talked about, but have a very important role to play — are called the pubo-coccygeus (pew-bo-kok-sij-ee-us) muscles.

Let's call them the PC muscles. They are located above and between your legs across the floor of your pelvis. They provide all the pelvic contractions used to retain your urine, bowel release and orgasms. They can bring more pleasure to you and your partner during sexual intercourse. When these muscles are toned up, your sexual sensations are heightened.

Childbirth and menopause can weaken these muscles, causing incontinence. Operations in the lower pelvic area can cause incontinence for both men and women. Have you experienced uncontrolled leakage when you laugh, cough, sneeze or have an orgasm? Then, take heart, you can strengthen those muscles by doing exercises developed by a gynecologist, Dr. Arnold Kegel, called, logically, the *Kegel* exercises.

In order to understand where the PC muscles are, sit on a toilet (for safety). As you relax, the urine will start to flow. Stop that flow with your muscles — not by crossing your legs or contracting your stomach muscles. Keep your focus on the muscles that squeeze off the flow. Those same muscles can stop a bowel movement and are also the muscles that contract and release during an orgasm.

Women have the advantage of being able to identify these muscles from the inside by inserting two fingers (well-lubricated) into the vagina and squeezing.

The Kegel Exercises

You can do these exercises sitting, standing or lying down — anywhere and at any time. They should be done at least three times a day. If you want to speed up recovering your strength there, do them as often as you can throughout the day.

❖ Squeeze your PC muscles — hold for a count of 5.

❖ Then relax. Repeat this sequence 10 times.

As you gain strength, you can build the hold count to 10 or more — and the repetitions to 50 or more.

❖ Another Kegel exercise is to
squeeze and relax the
PC muscles at a rapid pace.

Don't be discouraged if your rhythm is irregular. With practice, you will gain control over your PC muscles. You will have greater peace of mind when you have no more incontinence. And you can use the exercises at will during your lovemaking. You will experience heightened sensations, and your partner will appreciate your new talent.

Now, in preparation for your stretches and exercises, you must be aware of the correct way to perform them.

Are you short of breath after only a ten minute walk, or twice around the floor with your dance partner? Then you are "out of shape."

Throughout any exercise and stretching program, you must breathe correctly and move in smooth, rhythmic movements. These are good tools to apply to your daily life.

Breathing is an essential function of life's force. It creates energy, relaxation, mind and body balancing, and cleansing. By learning to breathe properly, you can create a meditative state to relax your body — a euphoric state to lift your spirits — a power state to have more stamina — a state of well-being — even a healing state.

Are you short of breath after only a ten minute walk, or five minutes of exercise, or twice around the floor with your dance partner? Then you are "out of shape."

By being a shallow breather, who has never learned to fill your lungs to their full capacity, you short-change your body of the oxygen it needs to keep running full power all day long.

You are probably a shallow breather who has never learned to fill your lungs to their full capacity. By being a shallow breather, you shortchange your body of the oxygen it needs to keep running at full power all day long.

Most people don't realize that their lungs will fill up with as much air as the space their lungs have to expand. A person who has practiced building up their lung capacity knows that their whole body cavity, from their shoulders to the bottom of their pelvis, will expand as they take in air properly. I have seen singers inhale so deeply that their back, chest, sides, abdomen and lower back expand at least two inches.

Let's see why: the diaphragm, which lies horizontally below your ribs, separating your chest cavity from your abdomen, is a muscular membranous partition that pushes the air out of the lungs when it contracts. When it relaxes, it expands into the abdomen and the lungs fill with air automatically. It works somewhat like a bellows that sucks air in when it expands and pushes air out when it contracts. And it does all this as an involuntary reflex.

Your chest, back and abdomen can be trained to expand more and more, in order to allow more space for that air to come in.

However, your emotions and stress can alter the normal function of your breathing. For instance, when you are frightened, your heart beats faster and your breathing becomes shallow — or you may hold your breath. The same thing occurs when you are under stress or are overtired. When this happens, be sure to STOP and take a few deep breaths. You will be giving your body the oxygen it needs to function under stress.

Most people think breathing takes place only in the chest. They become chest breathers or shallow breathers, never completely filling their lungs to capacity.

Do you think that only your chest is involved in breathing? Do you work too hard, get too little air, and then wilt like a dying flower when the day is only half-done? Let's find out:

❖ Lie on your back on the floor.

❖ Place one hand on your chest, and the other hand on your abdomen.

❖ Relax and breathe in.

❖ Then breathe out.

If you feel only your chest rise and fall, you are a shallow breather. However, if you feel your abdomen rise and fall, you are one of the fortunate ones who is getting more power out of your lungs.

If you are a shallow, chest breather, you are going to have to retrain yourself to allow your lungs to expand in all directions, taking in the huge amounts of the fresh air that will fill your entire body with power. Here's how —

How To Breathe Correctly!

❖ Lie on your back on the floor.

❖ Rest one hand on your chest and one hand on your abdomen. (Picture your body as a huge balloon that fills with air, starting from your toes and gradually filling all the way up to your neck.)

❖ Relax and slowly, silently, begin counting as you breathe in through your nose.

❖ *Visualize the air going all the way down into your toes. Feel your hand on your abdomen rise as you breathe deeply into your pelvis, expanding the sides and back of your hips. Then continue breathing in until your chest also rises. Feel the sides of your ribs and back expanding.*

Do not let your shoulders rise — keep your whole body relaxed — and let the air fill you up.

❖ When you feel you cannot take in any more air, hold your breath for a count of 5.

❖ Then slowly let the air gently flow out past your lips as though you were keeping a feather in the air.

❖ Count silently as the air flows out.

❖ *Feel your chest go down first — then your abdomen. Feel your stomach get flatter and flatter as you tighten your muscles and force the balance of that air out of your imaginary balloon. Feel the emptiness in your lungs. Feel the emptiness in your stomach. Feel yourself almost gasping for air.*

❖ *Relax.* See how eager your lungs are to fill up with fresh air.

❖ See how breathing is so necessary and becomes such a pleasure.

How high did you count each time? To 5? To 10? It doesn't matter what your number was. Counting is used only as a starting point to build on.

Now you have it. The basic exercise for building your lung capacity is:

- Breathe in to a count of 5.
- Hold for a count of 5.
- Breathe out to a count of 5.
- Hold for a count of 5.

Each new day's goal is simple. As your lung capacity grows, increase the count on each of the three steps. Soon, you will be breathing this way without even thinking about it.

This is the kind of breathing I want you to develop.

Be sure to use this breathing whenever adversity comes your way, and you will find it so much easier to deal with the stress. As you breathe in, imagine nourishment and goodness flowing into your body on those waves of air. While you hold the air in, feel it healing your body. As you breathe it out, imagine poisons and bad energy flowing out of your body.

Equally important, you are going to make this breathing the foundation for every stretch and exercise you perform. Deep breathing will help you do this with more ease and safety and it will support your body when it needs strength.

Breathe in on an easy move and breathe out on the action moves. Let's practice that for a minute.

- ❖ Stand up. Place yourself at ease. Check your posture. Be sure that you are standing straight so you can take in the maximum amount of air. Make sure your knees are relaxed — not locked.

- ❖ Hold up your right hand. Make a fist and look at it. You are going to use that hand as a breathing tool, to discover how your breath can give you undreamed-of power and strength.

❖ As you breathe in, relax and allow your hand to open slowly as your whole body is filling with air.

❖ *When you breathe in, your muscles should relax!*

❖ Then, as you breathe out, slowly begin to close the fingers into a fist.

❖ *When you breathe out, your muscles should contract!*

❖ As you close the fingers more and more tightly, force more and more air out by tightening your stomach muscles.

❖ The harder you squeeze, the harder you blow out the air. Feel your muscles work with you.

❖ Feel the power that is created by contracting your muscles as you blow the air out.

❖ Pause for a count of 3. Then, relax as you slowly breathe in and open your fingers.

❖ Feel the tension drain out of your hand.

❖ Feel the air flow into your lungs, relaxing and nourishing your whole body.

Practice this about 5 or 6 times right now. This technique coordinates your body and your breath to give you the strength and energy you need to perform any task.

Remember: Breathe *into* your whole body. Breathe *out from* your whole body.

Discover for yourself that deep breathing is not only more beneficial than shallow breathing, but gives you far more daily power.

This breathing technique also works with the heart muscle when it has to pump harder. If you are out of breath when you walk fast or climb stairs — *stop!* Take a few deep breaths until you feel your body is back in control.

Use Only Smooth and Rhythmic Movements

This is a good rule to apply to all activities in your life. However, in stretches and exercises, it is imperative.

Fast movements can pull muscles, hurt your back or throw a joint out of place. Never force a stretch or overdo exercises to the point of pain. "No pain, no gain" is *not* in my vocabulary.

Instead, because you are encouraging your muscles to control your movements, they must be slow, smooth and rhythmic. The best teacher of smooth and rhythmic movement is a cat. Watch it stretch for a moment. It moves slowly and gracefully, giving its muscles their full stretch and control. No move is abrupt. There is no strain. Just smooth grace and focused, sensuous power.

Put on some of your favorite music and move in rhythm to it. Make these stretches and exercises fun. I call my workout time my "dancing sessions." One day, I feel very energetic and play rock music. Another day, I feel elegant and play classical music. If I feel romantic, I play love songs.

Add to that fun by visualizing what you will look and feel like in a few weeks. You are building a lifestyle of well-being.

Fast movements can pull muscles, hurt your back or throw a joint out of place. Never force a stretch or overdo exercises to the point of pain. "No pain, no gain" is *not* in my vocabulary.

Tips To Make Your Firming Program So Enjoyable You'll Look Forward To It Each Morning

1. Open the window for fresh air.

2. Wear a leotard or panty and t-shirt to allow free movements. Better yet, do your exercises in the nude!

3. Raise your arms above your head as you breathe deeply, filling your lungs with fresh oxygen. Lower your arms as you blow the air out. Do this 5 times to start your energy.

4. Visualize the body that you are aiming for. This is the body you will gently build for yourself in the weeks and months to come. This is your inevitable reward.

5. Move to the rhythm of music you like. The rhythm should not be too fast or too slow. This smoothly coordinates your movements and creates a continuous environment of pleasure.

6. Make steady, smooth, even movements — not jerky or bouncy. This develops grace — grace in controlling the exercise, and grace in every movement of your entire day.

7. Don't stop if you begin sweating. That sweat consists of fat and toxins leaving your body.

8. Perform each exercise as many times as you can *without* having your muscles ache. Each week you should be able to do more than the week before.

9. Slowly stretch your muscles for 3 or 4 minutes after a vigorous workout.

10. If your muscles become stiff or sore, take a warm, luxurious bath and lightly massage them in the water.

11. Have one rest day every week. This gives the muscles time to relax and grow used to the number of exercises.

12. Do your stretches every day and your exercises every other day. You will find the "kinks" will disappear even more quickly.

13. When exercising on the floor, place a pillow under your knees to ease the tension in your lower back. Also, a pillow or neckroll under your head will make you feel more comfortable, particularly if you have a cervical problem.

14. Keep a chart of your measurements. Take them the same day every week. You will be inspired as you see the measurements shrink.

15. *Remember, you are not competing with anyone. You are not trying to prove how good or fast you are. Respect your body for the precious gift it is, and respect it for where it is on the fitness ladder.*

Note: Check with your doctor before you start any aerobic or weight-bearing exercises to be sure you do not have any physical problems that would put you in jeopardy.

❖ *Never, never, push your body past that point of pain! When you feel pain, immediately back off!*

❖ A dull ache every now and then — yes.

❖ But a sharp pain — *never!*

The ultimate goal is to enjoy your routine so that your body will hunger for it every day. Soon your body will become addicted to it. You will feel your muscles "itching to be stretched."

If you lovingly take care of your body and do your daily routine with pleasure, you will be rewarded in many ways.

Stretches are wonderful to loosen up and energize the body. Start your day with them. Take a stretch break whenever you feel tense or stiff throughout the day. It is also important to stretch before and after exercising to prevent muscle aches.

Although I have given you the number of times to repeat or hold each stretch or exercise, do only as many repititions as you feel comfortable with. As your muscles strengthen, you will feel comfortable working more repetitions. Gradually increase the number as your muscles tell you to go ahead.

At each session, be sure to do at least one stretch and exercise for each part of your body. Then gradually add more as you gain more strength. *The more you do, the faster you progress.*

The ultimate goal is to enjoy your routine so that your body will hunger for it every day. Soon your body will become addicted to it. You will feel your muscles "itching to be stretched."

P.S. There is no penalty for doing all of my stretches and exercises just for the fun of it, or just because it feels good.

It's such a great feeling to make yourself more alive!

Here Are Three 15-Minute Programs For You To Follow

The Easy-To-Do-Program is for you if you lead an inactive lifestyle and are not used to stretching and exercising. These are also helpful to the handicapped. It is the Gateway to Your Second Youth.

The Intermediate Program is for you if you are very active and have fairly good muscle tone. You have performed the *Easy-To-Do-Program* with ease and are ready to move forward.

The Advanced Program is for you if you are very flexible and have very good muscle tone. You probably have done stretching and exercising off and on, but want to increase your stamina and firm up your body.

You are starting to build your Second Youth. Begin with *The Easy-To-Do-Program* and work your way towards the higher goals. Your body will tell you when you are ready to move to the next level.

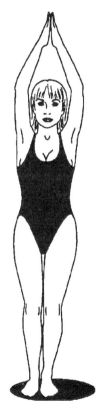

The Easy-To-Do-Program

Stretches

Stretch 1

- ❖ Stand with your feet 6 inches apart.
- ❖ Breathe in as you raise both arms over your head.
- ❖ Look up as you stretch towards the ceiling.
- ❖ Hold that stretch for a count of 5.

- ❖ Blow air out as you slowly lower your arms to your sides.
- ❖ Relax.
- ❖ Repeat this stretch 3 times in rhythm to music.

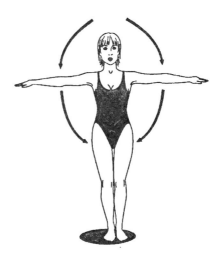

Stretch 2

- ❖ Stand with your feet 6 inches apart.
- ❖ Breathe in as you raise your right arm above your head.
- ❖ Place your left hand on your waist or thigh.
- ❖ Blow the air out as you slowly bend to the left.
- ❖ Hold for a count of 5.
- ❖ Breathe in as you return to an upright position. Lower both arms and relax.

REVERSE:

- ❖ Breathe in as you raise your left arm above your head.
- ❖ Place your right hand on your waist or thigh.
- ❖ Blow the air out as you slowly bend to the right.
- ❖ Hold for a count of 5.
- ❖ Breathe in as you return to the upright position.
- ❖ Lower both arms.
- ❖ Relax.
- ❖ Repeat this stretch 3 times in rhythm to slow music.

Stretch 3

- ❖ Still standing, with your feet 6 inches apart.
- ❖ Arms hanging by your sides — breathe in fully.
- ❖ Slowly blow the air out as your head drops to your chest.
- ❖ Bend your knees slightly and round your back.
- ❖ Gently bend down as far as you feel comfortable.
- ❖ Breathe normally as you hang there for a count of 5.
- ❖ Take a deep breath (knees still slightly bent).
- ❖ Blow the air out as you slowly *roll* your body up one vertebra at a time, starting from the bottom of your spine and ending with your head coming up last.
- ❖ Relax.
- ❖ Repeat this stretch 3 times in rhythm to slow music.

Stretch 4

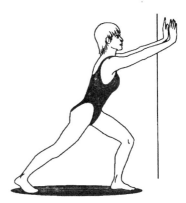

- ❖ Stand 1 to 2 feet from the wall, facing it.
- ❖ Put your hands on the wall.
- ❖ Bend your left knee and stretch your right foot back as far as you can so that only your toes touch the ground.
- ❖ Blow the air out as you slowly lower your right heel to the floor, pressing your hips forward. Feel the stretch in your calf muscle.
- ❖ Breathe in and relax — without changing your position.
- ❖ Now bend the knee of your right leg.

❖ Blow the air out as
you straighten your
left leg, moving your
hips backwards as
though you were
going to sit. Feel the
stretch behind your
left leg.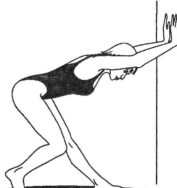

❖ Breathe in as you
come to a standing
position.

❖ Relax.

REVERSE:

❖ Put your hands on the wall.

❖ Bend your right knee and stretch your left foot back
as far as you can so that only your toes touch the
ground.

❖ Blow the air out as you slowly lower your left heel to
the floor, pressing your hips forward. Feel the stretch
in your calf muscle.

❖ Breathe in and relax — without changing your position.

❖ Now bend the knee of your left leg.

❖ Blow the air out as you straighten your right leg,
pressing your hips backwards as though you were
going to sit. Feel the stretch behind your right leg.

❖ Breathe in as you come to a standing position.

❖ Relax.

❖ Repeat this stretch 3 times.

Exercises

Underarms

* ❖ Sit or stand with feet 6 inches apart.
* ❖ Bend forward from your hips (back straight — not rounded).
* ❖ Hold your stomach muscles in to support your back.
* ❖ Keep your elbows next to your body at all times.
* ❖ Make fists, palms facing each other.
* ❖ Breathe in as you bring your fists towards your shoulders.
* ❖ Blow the air out as you *slowly* move your fists behind you.
* ❖ Repeat 10 times in rhythm to slow music.

Arms, Chest, Shoulders and Back

* ❖ Sit, stand or lie on the floor.
* ❖ Breathe in as you bring your arms out to your sides at shoulder level — do not bend your elbows.
* ❖ Blow the air out as you *slowly* bring your hands together in front — do not bend your elbows.
* ❖ Breathe in, then blow the air out as you press your hands together for a count of 5.
* ❖ Breathe in as you bring your arms back to your sides at shoulder level — pushing them back as far as possible as you lift your chest.
* ❖ Relax.
* ❖ Repeat 10 times in rhythm to music.

Waist and Stomach

❖ Lie on the floor.

❖ Rest your feet on a stool, chair or bed so your legs are bent in an upside down L shape. This will protect your back.

❖ Rest your hands by your side, and take a deep breath,

❖ Tighten your stomach muscles towards your back.

❖ Blow the air out as you *slowly* raise your upper body, leading with your chin — hands reaching towards your knees.

❖ This is an isometric crunch, so it doesn't matter how little you curl up. You may only get your head off the floor. That's a start. *Concentrate on your stomach muscles working.* As your muscles strengthen, you will automatically go higher.

❖ Breathe in as you *slowly* roll down.

❖ Relax.

❖ Repeat 10 times in rhythm to music.

Waist and Hips

❖ Lie on the floor, arms out to your sides at shoulder level.

❖ Raise your right knee towards your chest.

❖ Roll your head to the right.

❖ Shoulders and arms stay on the floor at all times.

❖ Breathe in and tighten your stomach muscles.

❖ Blow the air out as you *slowly* roll your hips and right knee towards the floor on your left side. (Go only as far as your body allows without pain.)

❖ Breathe in as you relax in that position to a count of 5.

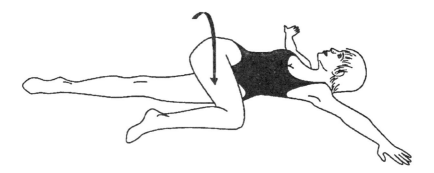

* Blow the air out as you *slowly* roll your hips and right knee back to starting position.
* Lower your leg and relax.

REVERSE:

* Raise your left knee towards your chest.
* Roll your head to the left.
* ***Shoulders and arms stay on the floor at all times.***
* Breathe in and tighten your stomach muscles.
* Blow the air out as you *slowly* roll your hips and left knee towards the floor on your right side. (Go only as far as your body allows without pain.)
* Breathe in as you relax in that position to a count of 5.
* Blow the air out as you *slowly* roll your hips and knee back to starting position.
* Lower your leg and relax.
* Repeat 10 times in rhythm to music.

Lower Abdomen, Buttocks, Thighs And Saddlebags

❖ Lie on the floor — arms at your sides.

❖ Bend knees and place your feet about 12 inches from your buttocks.

❖ Feet should be 6 inches apart, knees together.

❖ *Your shoulders, back and waist stay on the floor at all times. This will protect your lower back muscles.*

❖ Blow the air out as you tilt your pelvis up.

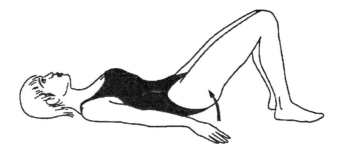

❖ Be sure you are tightening your stomach muscles towards your back.

❖ Squeeze your buttocks muscles together.

❖ Squeeze your knees together.

❖ Hold that squeeze for a count of 5.

❖ *Feel the muscles working from your waist down to your knees.*

❖ Breathe in and relax.

❖ Repeat 10 times in rhythm to music.

Outer Thighs (Saddlebags), Waist (Spare Tire)

NOTE: When doing this exercise, raise your leg only as far as your body will allow. Remember, you are not competing with anyone. As you grow stronger, you will go further. The slow movements are to strengthen the muscles and prevent injury.

- ❖ Lie on the floor on your left side.
- ❖ Rest your head on your left arm.
- ❖ Place your right hand on the floor in front of you.
- ❖ Bend your left leg to give you more balance.

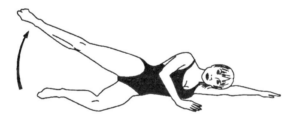

- ❖ Your right hand and left leg form a tripod for balance.
- ❖ Your right leg is straight.
- ❖ Blow the air out, tightening the stomach muscles, as you *slowly* raise your right leg.
- ❖ Breathe in as you hold your right leg up for a count of 5.
- ❖ Blow the air out as you *slowly* lower your leg to the floor.
- ❖ Repeat 10 times in rhythm to music.

REVERSE

* Lie on the floor on your right side.
* Rest your head on your right arm.
* Place your left hand on the floor in front of you.
* Bend your right leg.
* Your left leg is straight.
* Blow the air out, tightening the stomach muscles, as you *slowly* raise your left leg.
* Breathe in as you hold your left leg up for a count of 5.
* Blow the air out as you *slowly* lower your leg to the floor.
* Repeat 10 times in rhythm to music.

Stomach, Buttocks, Thighs, Calves, Ankles and Feet

* Stand, facing the back of a chair or whatever is waist high that you can hold onto for balance — feet together.
* Blow the air out, tightening your stomach and buttocks.
* *Slowly* raise your body to the tip of your toes. Hold for a count of 5 as you take in a deep breath.
* Then blow the air out as you *slowly* lower your heels back to the floor and relax.
* Repeat 10 times in rhythm to music.

Additional Stretches

Here are some additional stretches that I find very beneficial. You might want to exchange some or add them to your daily sessions. Also, throughout your day, you might find the need to use them for a particular part of your body.

To Open Your Chest and Relax Your Back

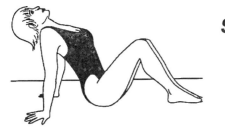

Stretch 1

❖ Sit on the floor with your knees bent.

❖ Place your hands slightly behind you at your sides to support the weight of your body.

❖ Breathe in deeply as you lean backward (arching your back).

❖ Raise your chin towards the ceiling and squeeze your shoulders back.

❖ *Feel the stretch across your chest and in your neck.*

❖ Then, breathe out as you bring your chin to your chest.

❖ Rock back on your hips and round your shoulders forward.

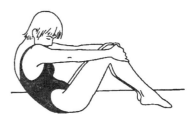

❖ Take a deep breath in that position.

❖ Feel the stretch across your shoulders and in your back.

❖ Relax.

❖ Repeat 5 times in rhythm to slow music.

Note: This stretch is also beneficial for asthmatic and bronchial conditions. It releases the tension in your chest and back muscles.

Stretch 2

- ❖ Lift your shoulders up to your ears and hold for a few seconds, then relax.

- ❖ *Slowly* roll your shoulders in circles forward 5 times, then backward 5 times.

- ❖ Now, *slowly* roll your shoulders forward alternating one at a time, 5 times.

- ❖ Reverse and alternately roll them backward 5 times.

Additional Exercises

Below are some additional exercises you can add to your daily session or do on alternate days.

Inner Thigh and Stomach

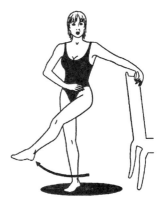

- ❖ Stand, holding back of chair or table for balance.

- ❖ Tighten your stomach muscles.

- ❖ Blow the air out as you *slowly* swing your left leg (foot flexed) across the front of your right leg.

- ❖ Hold for a count of 5 as you breathe in.

- ❖ Blow the air out as you *slowly* bring your left leg back to the left side (like a pendulum).

- ❖ Return your leg to the floor and relax.

- ❖ Repeat 10 times in rhythm to music.

Reverse

- ❖ Swing your right leg across the front of your left leg.

The Intermediate Program
Stretches
Stretch 1

- ❖ Stand with your feet 6 inches apart, arms at your sides.
- ❖ Breathe in and look up as you stretch upward with both arms.
- ❖ Stand on your toes and try to touch the ceiling.
- ❖ Hold that stretch for a count of 5.
- ❖ Blow the air out as you slowly lower your arms and heels.
- ❖ Relax.
- ❖ Repeat this stretch 5 times.

Stretch 2

In this stretch it is important to support your back by holding your stomach muscles in tightly and squeezing your buttocks.

- ❖ Stand with your feet 6 inches apart.
- ❖ Breathe in as you raise your arms over your head.
- ❖ Blow the air out as you *slowly* bend to the left.
- ❖ Hold for a count of 5, stomach muscles pulled in.
- ❖ Breathe in as you return to an upright position.
- ❖ Lower both arms.
- ❖ Relax.

REVERSE

- ❖ Breathe in as you raise your arms over your head.
- ❖ Blow the air out as you *slowly* bend to the right.
- ❖ Hold for a count of 5, stomach muscles pulled in.
- ❖ Breathe in as you return to the upright position.
- ❖ Lower both arms.
- ❖ Relax.
- ❖ Repeat this stretch 5 times.

Stretch 3

- ❖ Stand with your feet 6 inches apart, arms hanging by your sides — breathe in fully.
- ❖ *Slowly* blow the air out as you let your head drop to your chest.
- ❖ Bend your knees slightly and round your back.
- ❖ Gently bend down until your hands reach the floor (or wherever you feel most comfortable without pain).
- ❖ *Slowly* straighten your legs.
- ❖ Breathe normally as you hang there for a count of 5.
- ❖ Take a deep breath, *slightly bend your knees* to take the pressure off your back.
- ❖ Blow the air out *slowly* as you *roll* your body up — one vertebra at a time — starting from the bottom and ending with your head coming up last.
- ❖ Take in a deep breath and relax.
- ❖ Repeat this stretch 5 times.

Stretch 4

- ❖ Stand 1 to 2 ft. from a wall, facing it.

- ❖ Put your hands on the wall.

- ❖ Bend your left knee and stretch your right foot back as far as you can so that only your toes touch the ground.

- ❖ Blow the air out as you *slowly* lower your right heel to the floor, pressing your hips forward. Feel the stretch in your calf muscle. (Press your hips forward harder for a deeper stretch.)

- ❖ Breathe in and relax — without changing your position.

- ❖ Now, bend the knee of your right leg.

- ❖ Blow the air out as you straighten your left leg, pressing your hips backwards as though you were going to sit. (The more you press your hips backward, the deeper the stretch in the back of your leg will be.)

- ❖ Breathe in as you come to a standing position.

- ❖ Relax.

REVERSE

- ❖ Put your hands on the wall.

- ❖ Bend your right knee and stretch your left foot back as far as you can so that only your toes touch the ground.

- ❖ Blow the air out as you slowly lower your left heel to the floor, pressing your hips forward.

- ❖ Breathe in and relax — without changing your position.

- ❖ Now bend the knee of your left leg.

- ❖ Blow the air out as you straighten your right leg, pressing your hips backwards as though you were going to sit.

- ❖ Breathe in as you come to a standing position and relax.

- ❖ Repeat 5 times.

Exercises

When I mention *weights,* start with 2 lbs. and work up to 3 lbs. or more. You can find them in any sports store. Use free weights (hand held), wrist weights, or ankle weights. You can substitute books, cans, or whatever you create from your household.

When I mention *stretcher,* that also can be found in a sports store. You can substitute an elastic belt, rubber hose, bicycle inner tube, twisted towel, or any device you can pull on to give you isometric tension.

Back of Arms (Underarms)

❖ Use 2 lb. weights in your hands or on your wrists.

❖ Sit or stand with feet 6 inches apart.

❖ Bend forward from your hips (back straight — not rounded).

❖ Hold your stomach muscles in to support your back.

❖ Keep your elbows next to your body at all times.

❖ Breathe in as you bring your hands towards your shoulders.

❖ Blow the air out as you slowly move your hands behind you.

❖ Repeat 10 times in rhythm to slow music.

Arms, Chest, Shoulders and Back

❖ Use 2 lb. weights in your hands or on your wrists.

❖ Sit, stand or lie on the floor.

❖ Breathe in as you bring your arms out to your sides at shoulder level — do not bend your elbows.

❖ Blow the air out as you *slowly* bring your hands together in front — do not bend your elbows.

❖ Breathe in, then blow the air out as you press your hands together for a count of 5.

❖ Breathe in as you bring your arms back to your sides at shoulder level — pushing them back as far as possible as you lift your chest.

❖ Relax.

❖ Repeat 10 times in rhythm to music.

Waist and Stomach

❖ Lie on the floor, knees bent, or . . .

❖ Rest your feet on a stool, chair or bed so your legs are bent in an upside down L shape. This will protect your back.

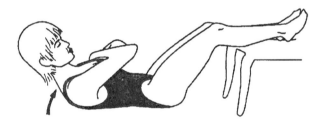

❖ Cross your arms over your chest, or clasp each elbow with the opposite hand.

❖ Breathe in as you tighten your stomach muscles.

❖ Blow the air out as you *slowly* raise your upper body.

❖ Concentrate on your stomach muscles doing the work.

❖ If you can't raise your shoulders off the floor, that's OK. The stomach muscles are getting their workout no matter how far you go.)

❖ Breathe in as you *slowly* return to the floor.

❖ Relax.

❖ Repeat 10 times in rhythm to music.

Waist, Hip and Side Muscles

❖ Lie on the floor, arms out to your sides at shoulder level.

❖ Raise your right knee towards your chest.

❖ Roll your head to the right.

❖ *Shoulders and arms stay on the floor at all times.*

❖ Breathe in and tighten your stomach muscles.

❖ Blow the air out as you *slowly* roll your hips and right knee towards the floor on your left side. (Go only as far as your body allows without pain.)

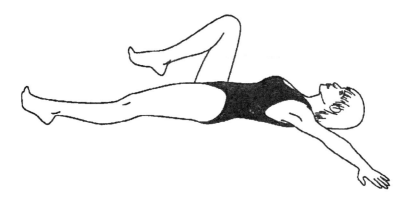

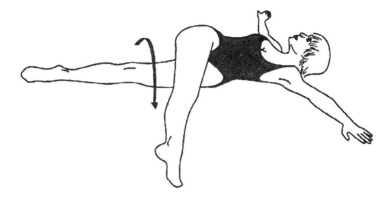

❖ Straighten your right leg and *slowly* stretch in the twist.

❖ Bend your right leg and breathe in as you relax in that position to a count of 5.

❖ Blow the air out as you *slowly* roll your hips and right knee back to starting position.

❖ Lower your leg and relax.

REVERSE:

❖ Raise your left knee towards your chest.

❖ Roll your head to the left.

❖ *Shoulders and arms stay on the floor at all times.*

❖ Breathe in and tighten your stomach muscles.

❖ Blow the air out as you *slowly* roll your hips and left knee towards the floor on your right side. (Go only as far as your body allows without pain.)

❖ Straighten your left leg and *slowly* stretch in the twist.

❖ Bend your left leg and breathe in as you relax in that position for a count of 5.

❖ Blow the air out as you *slowly* roll your hips and left knee back to starting position.

❖ Lower your leg and relax.

❖ Repeat 10 times in rhythm to music.

Lower Abdomen, Lower Back, Buttocks, Thighs And Saddlebags

If you have back problems, check with your doctor before you try this exercise.

❖ Lie on the floor — arms at your sides — palms down.

❖ Bend your knees and place your feet about 12 inches from your buttocks.

❖ Your feet should be 6 inches apart, knees together.

❖ *Shoulders and upper back stay on the floor at all times.*

❖ Blow the air out as you raise your pelvis.

❖ *Be sure you are tightening your stomach muscles towards your back.*

❖ Squeeze your buttocks muscles together.

❖ Squeeze your knees together.

❖ Hold that squeeze for a count of 5.

❖ *Feel the muscles working from your waist down to your knees.*

❖ Breathe in and relax.

❖ Repeat 10 times in rhythm to music.

Outer Thighs (Saddlebags), Waist (Spare Tire)

When doing this exercise, raise your leg only as far as your body will allow. You are not competing with anyone. As you grow stronger, you will go further. The slow movements are to strengthen the muscles and prevent injury.

❖ Put a 2 lb. ankle weight on each ankle.

❖ Lie on the floor on your left side.

❖ Rest your head on your left arm.

❖ Place your right hand on the floor in front of you.

❖ Bend your left leg to give you more balance. (Your right hand and left leg form a tripod for balance.)

❖ Your right leg is straight. Blow the air out, tightening your stomach muscles.

❖ *Slowly* raise your right leg.

❖ Breathe in as you hold your right leg up for a count of 5.

❖ Blow the air out as you *slowly* lower your leg to an inch above the floor. (You will gain better muscle control if you do not let your leg go all the way to the floor.)

❖ Be sure your body is straight and your stomach muscles are supporting your back.

❖ Repeat 10 times in rhythm to music.

REVERSE:

❖ Lie on the floor on your right side.

❖ Rest your head on your right arm.

❖ Place your right hand on the floor in front of you.

❖ Bend your right leg to give you more balance.

❖ Your left leg is straight.

❖ Blow the air out, tightening the stomach muscles.

❖ *Slowly* raise your left leg.

❖ Breathe in as you hold your left leg up for a count of 5.

❖ Blow the air out as you *slowly* lower your leg to an inch above the floor.

❖ Repeat 10 times in rhythm to music.

Stomach, Buttocks, Thighs, Calves, Ankles and Feet

❖ Stand beside a chair or whatever is waist high for balance. Place both hands on that support — feet together.

❖ Blow the air out, tightening your stomach and buttocks.

❖ *Slowly* raise your body to the tips of your toes.

❖ Hold for a count of 5 as you take in a deep breath.

❖ Then blow the air out as you *slowly* lower your heels and your body to a squatting position.

❖ *At all times, the trunk of your body must remain straight.*

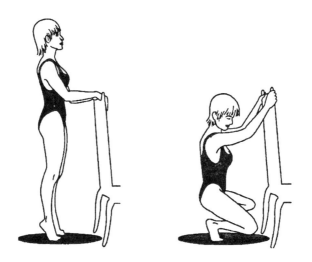

- ❖ Breathe in and relax in that position for a count of 5.
- ❖ Blow the air out, tightening your stomach and buttocks.
- ❖ Raise your body back to a standing position.
- ❖ Breathe in and relax.
- ❖ Repeat 10 times in rhythm to music.

Additional Stretches

Here are additional stretches that I feel are very beneficial. You might want to exchange or add some to your daily sessions. Also, at different times throughout your day, you might feel the need to stretch a particular area of your body.

Stretch 1

- ❖ Lie on your back and bring your knees up towards your chest.
- ❖ Stretch your arms out on the floor at shoulder level — both shoulders remain on the floor at all times.
- ❖ Rock your lower torso from side to side.
- ❖ Then let your knees roll to your right side, and your head to your left.
- ❖ Relax in that position and breathe naturally.
- ❖ Roll back onto your back, knees towards your chest.
- ❖ Roll your knees to the left side, and your head to the right.
- ❖ Relax in that position and breathe naturally.
- ❖ Roll back onto your back, knees towards your chest.
- ❖ Lower your legs and relax.

This will massage the muscles in your back.

Stretch 2

- ❖ Lie on your back, bring your knees up towards your chest.

- ❖ Place your hands on your knees or wrap your knees with your arms.

- ❖ Rock backwards and forwards as though you were in a rocking chair.

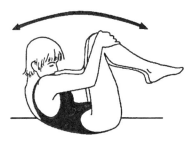

Stretch 3

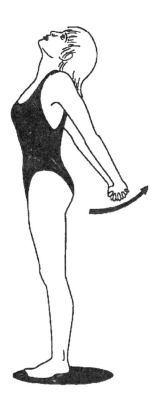

- ❖ Sit or stand with feet apart.

- ❖ Breathe in as you clasp your hands behind you.

- ❖ Blow the air out as you *slowly* raise your clasped hands behind you, keeping your shoulders relaxed and tilting your head back.

- ❖ Repeat 10 times in rhythm to music.

Anytime throughout the day, this is a wonderful stretch to relieve the tension that builds up in your shoulders and back.

Additional Exercises

❖ Here are some additional exercises that you might want to exchange or add to your sessions.

Front of Arms

- ❖ Put 2 lb. weights in your hands or on your wrists.
- ❖ Sit or stand with your feet apart.
- ❖ Arms at your sides, palms facing front.
- ❖ Blow the air out as you *slowly* lift your hands to your shoulders.
- ❖ Breathe in as you *slowly* lower them back to your sides.
- ❖ Repeat 10 times in rhythm to music.

Front of Arms and Chest

- ❖ Sit or stand with feet apart or you can lie on the floor.
- ❖ With a stretcher in your hands, hold arms in front of you at shoulder level, palms *down*.
- ❖ Blow the air out as you *slowly* pull your hands apart.
- ❖ Breathe in as you bring them together.
- ❖ Repeat 10 times in rhythm to music.
- ❖ 2 lb. weights can be used instead of a stretcher.

Arms, Back and Shoulders (Widow's Hump)

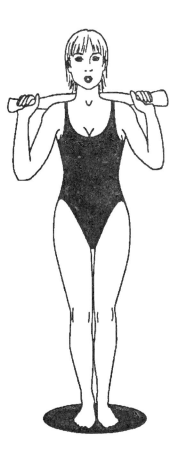

❖ Sit or stand with feet apart.

❖ Put a stretcher in your hands, palms facing down.

❖ Breathe in as you raise your arms above your head, pulling your hands apart.

❖ Blow the air out as you *slowly* lower the stretcher behind your head, still pulling your hands apart. (Feel the squeeze in your shoulders and upper back).

❖ Breathe in as you raise them again and lower your hands in front of you.

❖ Relax.

❖ Repeat 10 times in rhythm to music.

Waist And Stomach

❖ Lie on the floor — rest your feet on a stool, chair or bed so that your legs are bent in an upside down L shape.

❖ Cross your arms over your chest, or clasp each elbow with the opposite hand.

❖ Take a deep breath and tighten your stomach muscles towards your back as you blow the air out.

❖ *Without taking a breath in*, raise your upper body, leading with your chin.

❖ Concentrate on the tightening of your stomach muscles as you raise your upper body.

❖ Breathe in as you *slowly* roll your body back down.

❖ Relax.

❖ Repeat 10 times in rhythm to music.

❖ As your strength allows, you can increase the number of repeats.

Stomach Lift

This exercise should be done throughout the day wherever you may be (sitting, standing, walking, or lying down).

❖ Take a deep breath and tighten your stomach muscles as you blow all of the air out.

❖ *Without taking a breath in*, contract your stomach muscles, lifting your ribs and chest off your hips (shoulders relaxed) and hold for a count of 10.

❖ Breathe in as you relax.

❖ Repeat 10 times.

❖ You will feel your body straightening and your inner muscles strengthening to hold your inner organs in place.

Another Extension of The Stomach Lift

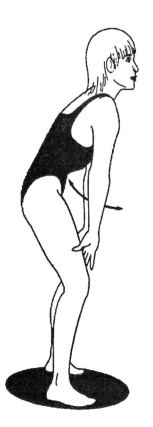

❖ Stand with your hands resting just above your knees.

❖ Slightly bend your legs to take the stress off your back.

❖ Blow all the air out and tighten your stomach muscles.

❖ Draw the stomach muscles up and in, forming a hollow. (Feel the internal muscles lift your organs and stomach.)

❖ *Do not inhale while this lift is being maintained.*

❖ Push your stomach muscles in and out until you feel the need to breathe again.

You will see a great cavity between your ribs and get a real sense of how much control you can exercise over your internal muscles.

This is an exercise in yoga that works very well to strengthen the muscles that hold the organs in place.

Inner Thigh and Stomach

❖ Lie on the floor on your back.

❖ Place your hands or a pillow under your hips to protect the muscles in your lower back.

❖ Bend your knees, then raise your legs straight up in the air.

❖ Tighten your stomach muscles and squeeze your buttocks.

❖ Breathe in as you *slowly* spread your legs out to the sides.

❖ Hold for a count of 5 as you breathe comfortably.

❖ Blow the air out as you *slowly* bring your legs back to the straight up position.

❖ Repeat 10 times in rhythm to music.

The Advanced Program

Stretches

Stretch 1

❖ Stand with feet 6 inches apart, arms at sides.

❖ Clasp your hands behind you.

❖ Squeeze your buttocks and tighten your stomach muscles.

❖ Lift your chest and look up towards the ceiling as you breathe in, raising your clasped hands as far as possible.

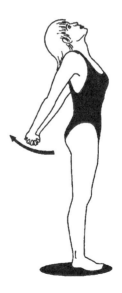

❖ Hold for a count of 5. Feel the stretch across your chest, shoulders and neck. Feel the squeeze in the muscles of your back.

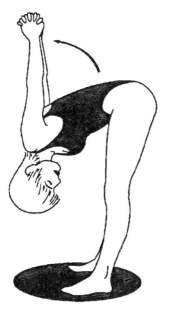

❖ Blow the air out as you bend forward, hands still clasped behind you, raising them as high as possible.

❖ Feel the stretch in your back and behind your legs.

❖ Hang there for a count of 5, breathing normally.

❖ Blow the air out as you raise your torso, vertebra by vertebra, head coming up last.

❖ Relax your arms and breathe in.

❖ Repeat 10 times in rhythm to music.

Stretch 2

❖ Sitting on the floor, extend your right leg in front.

❖ Bring your left foot to rest on the side of your right leg as far above your knee as is comfortable.

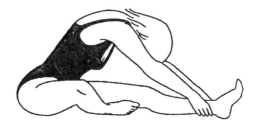

❖ Breathe in as you raise your hands above your head.

❖ Turn your body towards your right leg.

❖ Blow the air out as you lower your body over your right leg.

❖ Place your hands on your right leg, as far down as you feel comfortable. Put your head down between your arms.

❖ Relax in that position, letting your torso and leg muscles stretch, without pain, as you breathe naturally for a count of 5.

❖ As you breathe into your leg, you will find your muscles relaxing with each breath.

❖ If you feel you can stretch even farther, bend your elbows, bringing your body closer to your leg.

❖ Blow the air out as you *slowly* raise your torso, vertebra by vertebra — head coming up last.

❖ *If your back and stomach muscles are strong enough, you can begin your torso raise with your arms stretched above your head. Then the body is raised as one unit from the hip, with a flat back.*

REVERSE

❖ Left leg extended in front.

❖ Right foot on the side of the left leg as far above the knee as is comfortable.

❖ Breathe in as you raise your arms above your head.

❖ Turn your body towards your left leg.

❖ Blow the air out as you lean forward over your legs until you can place your hands on the outstretched leg comfortably.

❖ Relax in that position as you count to 5.

❖ If you feel you can stretch even farther, bend your elbows, bringing your body closer to your leg.

❖ Blow the air out as you *slowly* raise your torso, vertebra by vertebra — head coming up last.

❖ *If your back and stomach muscles are strong enough, you can begin your torso raise with your arms stretched above your head. Then the body is raised as one unit from the hip, with a flat back.*

❖ Stretch both legs out and bounce them on the floor to massage the muscles.

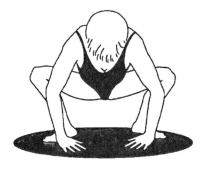

Stretch 3

❖ Sit in a squatting position, feet about 12 inches apart.

❖ Place your hands on the floor in front of you.

❖ Elbows should touch your inner knees.

❖ Lean your torso forward slightly for balance.

❖ Blow the air out as you press your knees out with your elbows. Feel the stretch in your inner thigh and your lower back.

❖ You can place your feet at different distances apart to find the position that is right for you.

Stretch 4

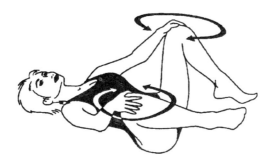

- ❖ Lie on your back.

- ❖ Bring your knees up towards your chest.

- ❖ Hold them with your hands or arms, while breathing naturally. This will release your back muscles and stretch them out.

- ❖ With your right hand on your right knee and your left hand on your left knee, make circles in the air.

- ❖ First clockwise — then counter-clockwise.

- ❖ Then circle each knee in opposite directions.

- ❖ Lower your legs and relax.

Exercises

When I mention *weights*, start with 3 lbs. and work up to 5 lbs. or more. Use free weights (hand held), wrist weights or ankle weights. You can substitute books, cans, or whatever you create from your household. However, when using the heavier weights, it is preferable to use the weights found in any sports store. They are designed to wrap around your wrists and ankles or be held in your hands more easily. There is less risk of hurting yourself.

When I mention *stretcher*, that also can be found in a sports store. You can substitute an elastic belt, rubber hose, bicycle inner tube, twisted towel, or any device you can pull on that will give you isometric tension.

Back of Arms (Underarms)

❖ Use 3 lb. weights in your hands or on your wrists.

❖ Sit or stand with feet 6 inches apart.

❖ Hold your stomach muscles in to support your back.

❖ Raise hands towards the ceiling, palms facing behind you.

❖ Breathe in as you bend your arms at the elbows and lower your hands towards your shoulders.

❖ Blow the air out as you lift your hands towards the ceiling.

❖ Repeat 10 times in rhythm to slow music.

Arms, Chest, Shoulders and Back

❖ Use 3 lb. weights in your hands or on your wrists.

❖ Sit or stand with feet apart, or you can lie on the floor.

❖ Raise your arms out to the sides at shoulder level, palms facing forward.

❖ Blow the air out as you *slowly* bring your hands together in front of you, without bending your elbows.

❖ Breathe in as you return them to your sides at shoulder level, without bending your elbows.

❖ Repeat 10 times in rhythm to music.

NOTE: This exercise uses many muscles in your upper body, so be sure to move *slowly* and feel the muscles working.

Waist, Spare Tire, Upper Hip and Stomach

Note: If you feel your muscles straining, you can do this exercise with less weight in your hands or with no weights at all. The weight of your raised arms will be heavy enough. If holding both arms up creates too much weight, you can do the same exercise with one arm up and the other resting on your waist or thigh.

❖ Use 3 lb. weights in each hand or use wrist weights.

❖ Stand with feet 6 inches apart.

❖ Pull your stomach muscles in to support your back and tighten your buttocks. (It is very important to maintain this posture throughout the whole exercise.)

❖ Breathe in as you raise your hands towards the ceiling.

❖ Blow the air out as you lift your upper body and *slowly* bend to your left side, making sure your body does not twist. Your body should face the front at all times.

❖ Hold for a count of 5.

❖ Breathe in as you *slowly* straighten up, hands stretching towards the ceiling.

❖ Then, blow the air out as you lift your upper body and *slowly* bend to the right side.

❖ Hold for a count of 5.

❖ Breathe in as you *slowly* straighten up.

❖ Lower your arms to your sides and relax.

❖ Repeat 10 times in rhythm to slow music.

Lower Abdomen, Back, Buttocks, Thighs and Saddlebags

Note: If you have back problems, check with your doctor before you try this exercise.

* ❖ Lie on the floor — arms at your sides.
* ❖ Bending your knees, place your feet 6 inches apart and 12 inches from your buttocks.
* ❖ Breathe in and press your knees together.
* ❖ Blow the air out as you lift your pelvis towards the ceiling.

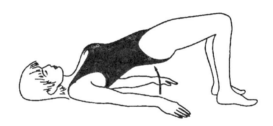

* ❖ *Shoulders stay on the floor at all times.*
* ❖ Hold your stomach muscles in and squeeze your buttocks tightly as you open and close your knees *slowly* 10 times.
* ❖ *Feel the muscles working in your lower abdomen, buttocks, back and thighs.*
* ❖ Breathe in and relax *slowly* to the floor.
* ❖ Repeat 10 times in rhythm to music.

NOTE: You can work different muscles in your thighs by spreading your feet farther apart or by placing them next to each other.

Outer Thighs (Saddlebags), Waist (Spare Tire)

Note: Raise your leg only as far as your body will allow. You are not competing with anyone. As you grow stronger, you will go further. **Do not swing your leg** or the force of the uncontrolled momentum might injure your hip or pull a muscle.

- Use 3 lb. ankle weights.
- Stand holding the back of a chair or a table.
- Stand tall and breathe in.
- Blow the air out as you *slowly* raise your right leg to the side.
- Hold for a count of 5 as you breathe in.
- Then blow the air out as you *slowly* lower your right leg.
- Repeat 10 times in rhythm to music.

REVERSE YOUR POSITION

- Stand tall and breathe in — tighten your stomach muscles.
- Blow the air out as you *slowly* raise your left leg to the side.
- Hold for a count of 5 as you breathe in.
- Then blow the air out as you *slowly* lower your left leg.
- Repeat 10 times in rhythm to music.

Back Of Thighs, Buttocks, and Stomach

This exercise can be done in three different positions. Choose which one feels right for you.

1. Stand, holding the back of a chair or table for balance.
2. Lie on the floor on your left side, head resting on your left arm, right hand on floor for balance, left knee bent.
3. Get on both hands and knees on the floor.

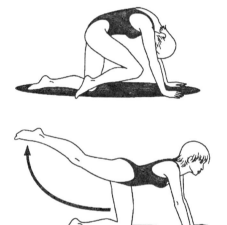

- ❖ Use 3 lb. ankle weights.

- ❖ Breathe in as you bring your right knee towards your chest.

- ❖ Tighten your stomach muscles to support your back.

- ❖ Blow the air out as you *slowly* bring your right leg straight out behind you, leading with your heel. Lift it only as high as you can without discomfort.

- ❖ Hold for a count of 5.

- ❖ Breathe in as you bring your knee back towards your chest.

- ❖ Repeat 10 times in rhythm to music.

REVERSE POSITIONS

❖ Breathe in as you bring your left knee towards your chest.

❖ Tighten your stomach muscles to support your back.

❖ Blow the air out as you *slowly* bring your left leg straight out behind you, leading with your heel.

❖ Hold for a count of 5.

❖ Breathe in as you bring your knee back towards your chest.

❖ Repeat 10 times in rhythm to music.

Additional Exercises

❖ Here are some additional exercises. You might want to exchange some in your morning session or do them on alternate days.

Front of Arms and Chest

❖ Sit or stand with feet apart. Or you can lie on the floor.

❖ With a stretcher in your hands, hold your arms at shoulder level, palms up.

❖ Blow the air out as you *slowly* pull your hands apart.

❖ Breathe in as you bring them together —

❖ Repeat 10 times in rhythm to music.

❖ 3 lb. weights can be used instead of a stretcher.

Back of Arms (Underarms)

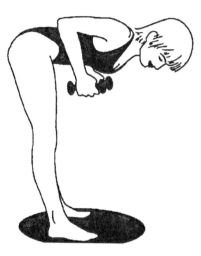

- ❖ Sit or stand with feet apart.

- ❖ Put a 3 lb. weight in each hand, arms by your sides, palms facing each other.

- ❖ Bend forward from your hips (keep your back straight — not rounded), making sure you hold your stomach muscles in to support your back.

❖ Breathe in as you bring your hands to your shoulders (keep your elbows close to your body).

- ❖ Blow the air out as you *slowly* extend your arms behind you.

- ❖ Breathe in as you bring your hands back towards your shoulders.

- ❖ Repeat 10 times in rhythm to music.

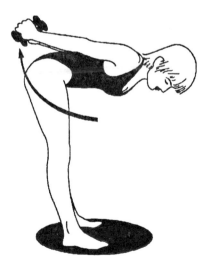

Waist, Spare Tire, Upper Hip

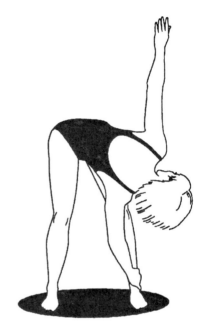

- ❖ Sit or stand with your feet 12 inches apart.

- ❖ *Keep your stomach muscles pulled in to support your back.*

- ❖ Breathe in as you raise your arms out to the side at shoulder level.

- ❖ Twist your upper body to the left, keeping your hips forward.

- ❖ Blow the air out as you *slowly* bend, touching your right hand to your left foot. Your left hand points to the ceiling — look towards your left hand.

- ❖ Breathe in as you straighten up and relax.

REVERSE

- ❖ Breathe in as you raise your arms out to the side at shoulder level.

- ❖ Twist your upper body to the right, keeping your hips forward.

- ❖ Blow the air out as you *slowly* bend, touching your left hand to your right foot. Your right hand points to the ceiling and you look towards your right hand.

- ❖ Breathe in as you straighten up and relax.

- ❖ Repeat 10 times in rhythm to music.

Waist (Spare Tire), Hips

❖ Lie on the floor — arms out to sides at shoulder level.

❖ Shoulders and arms stay on the floor at all times.

❖ Raise your right leg towards the ceiling.

❖ Roll your head to the right and breathe in.

❖ Blow the air out as you *slowly* roll your leg and hips to the left side.

❖ Breathe in as you relax in that position to a count of 5.

❖ Blow the air out as you *slowly* roll your leg and hips back to starting position.

❖ Lower your leg and relax.

REVERSE

❖ Raise your left leg towards the ceiling.

❖ Shoulders and arms are flat on the floor.

❖ Roll your head to the left and breathe in.

❖ Blow the air out as you *slowly* roll your leg and hips to the right side.

❖ Breathe in as you relax in that position to a count of 5.

❖ Blow the air out as you *slowly* roll your leg and hips back to starting position. Lower your leg and relax.

❖ Repeat this exercise 10 times in rhythm to music.

Inner Thigh, Stomach and Buttocks

* ❖ Lie on the floor on your left side.

* ❖ Rest your head on your left arm.

* ❖ Place your right hand on the floor in front of you for balance.

* ❖ Bending your right knee, place your right foot flat on the floor in front of you.

* ❖ *Your right hand and foot will give you leverage to lift your left leg.*

* ❖ Your left leg is lying straight in line with your body.

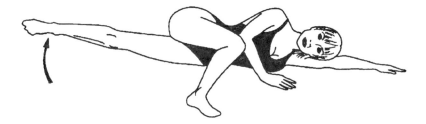

* ❖ Tighten your stomach muscles and squeeze your buttocks.

* ❖ Blow the air out as you lift your left leg (concentrate on the inner thigh muscles working to pull it up).

* ❖ Hold for a count of 5.

* ❖ Breathe in as you *slowly* return your left leg to the floor.

* ❖ Repeat 10 times in rhythm to music.

REVERSE

- ❖ Lie on your right side, head resting on your right arm.

- ❖ Place your left hand on the floor in front of you.

- ❖ Bending your left knee, place your left foot flat on the floor in front of you.

- ❖ Tighten your stomach muscles and squeeze your buttocks.

- ❖ Blow the air out as you lift your right leg.

- ❖ Hold for a count of 5.

- ❖ Breathe in as you *slowly* return your right leg to the floor.

Stomach, Buttocks, Thighs, Calves and Feet

- ❖ Stand, holding the back of a chair or a bar at waist level. Place your feet 12 inches apart.

- ❖ *At all times, your body must remain straight, your stomach and buttocks muscles must be held in tightly. Your legs, ankles and feet muscles are doing all the work.*

- ❖ Breathe in as you *slowly* raise your body to the tip of your toes.

- ❖ Blow the air out as you lower your buttocks to a squat position (still on the tip of your toes).

- ❖ Take a deep breath and relax in that position —

- ❖ Blow the air out as you raise your body back to a standing position.

- ❖ Relax your heels to the floor and breathe in.

- ❖ Repeat 10 times in rhythm to music.

NOTE: Different muscles can be activated by placing your feet farther apart.

Ankles and Toes

The most neglected part of your body!

❖ Exercise 1

- While sitting, raise your feet off the floor and rotate them by drawing imaginary circles in the air — first clockwise 10 times. Relax.

- Then rotate your feet counterclockwise 10 times. Relax.

❖ Exercise 2

- While sitting, point your toes and turn each foot to the right as though you were trying to reach for something with them.

- Hold for a count of 5. Relax.

- Then point your toes and turn each foot to the left.

- Hold for a count of 5. Relax.

❖ Exercise 3

- While sitting, tuck your toes under and place your feet under your chair as far back as you can.

- Then apply pressure downward, giving a stretch to the top of your feet. Hold for a count of 5. Relax.

❖ Exercise 4

- While sitting, hold your feet out in front of you.

- Curl your toes under tightly, then spread them apart.

- Repeat 10 times.

- Then shake your feet 10 times. Relax.

❖ Exercise 5

- Pick up objects with your toes — first with your right foot, then with your left foot.

- Repeat with each foot 5 times.

❖ Exercise 6

- Massage your feet and toes each morning and each evening. This will relieve stress throughout your body. Applying lotion or oil to your feet will make your hands glide over your skin more easily and a bonus will be softer feet without calluses.

Hands and Wrists

❖ Exercise 1

- Rotate your hands from the wrist by drawing circles in the air — first clockwise 10 times. Relax.

- Then rotate your hands counterclockwise 10 times. Relax.

❖ Exercise 2

- Curl your hands into fists and bend them towards your arms.

- Hold for a count of 5. Relax.

- Open your hands and with the right hand, bend your left hand backwards. Hold for a count of 5. Relax.

- With your left hand, bend your right hand backwards.

- Hold for a count of 5. Relax.

❖ **Exercise 3**

- Curl your hands into tight fists, then open your hands and spread your fingers as widely apart as possible.

- Repeat 10 times. Relax.

❖ **Exercise 4**

- Relax your hands and shake them vigorously 10 times.

❖ **Exercise 5**

- Apply hand lotion or massage oil to your hands.

- Massage each hand from the wrist up through each finger. Be sure to massage around each knuckle and finger joint on your hand.

- There are many pressure points in the palm of your hand. Be sure to massage every inch of it well, extending through to the tips of your fingers and thumb.

Ancient remedies for relieving stress and pain have been to massage the pressure points in the hands and feet that correspond to different organs and areas of the body. One of these is Reflexology and there are charts which show those pressure points and the parts of the body they correspond to. They can be found in bookstores (particularly those specializing in oriental and natural healing). You should try it! You will be amazed at how good it makes you feel!

Tension Releasing Exercise

This exercise can be repeated throughout the day while standing or sitting at your desk.

❖ Blow the air out, tightening your buttocks and stomach muscles.

❖ Squeeze your knees together and press your pelvis forward.

❖ Relax and breathe in, still holding your muscles tightly. Blow the air out as you *slowly* bend over towards the floor.

❖ Hang there for a count of 10 while you breathe normally.

❖ Blow the air out as you *slowly* raise your body (vertebra by vertebra) back to the upright position. Your head comes up last.

The stress in the small of your back, shoulders and neck will be relieved and you will feel renewed energy flow throughout your body.

NOTE: When you sneeze, cough, bend over or lift heavy objects, be sure to tighten the stomach and buttocks muscles. This will protect you from muscle strain and stress on the lower back.

Once you have reached your goal of well-being, you can maintain your strength and shape with just a couple of sessions a week. But be aware that giving up and returning to a sedentary life will signal your body to go back to its aging process.

You can substitute the workout sessions with activities you might enjoy doing with other people or alone — activities such as bicycling, swimming, climbing mountains, dancing, long fast walks, playing tennis, etc. An active life is very rewarding and rich in all the pleasures of living.

Your body is miraculous in its tenacity and healing powers.

The more you care for your body, the more responsive it will be. This care includes exercise, massage, trager, reflexology, yoga, or any other kind of activity in motion.

The Rewards Are There For You — You Only Have To Apply Yourself.

23

Face Exercises, Skin Care and Makeup: How To Have a More Beautiful Face than You Had As a Young Woman

Since I started in the modeling and beauty business — amazingly enough, a total of over 35 years — I have deliberately collected all the proven beauty secrets I could find from my professional model friends and the cosmetic companies I worked for.

I realize that heredity does have something to do with what you look like, but I firmly believe anyone can enhance their individual beauty. I feel even more strongly that you can work with Mother Nature to prevent Father Time from making his mark on your appearance.

STEP ONE: FACIAL EXERCISES

Your face has many muscles that respond to the repetitive movements you put them through in your daily expressions. Wrinkles and sagging muscles can be reversed. You can firm your face just as you firm your body. You can look younger. You can look *better* than you did when you were younger.

If you are over 50 and already have sagging jowls and wrinkles due to sun-damage, smoking, drinking, or poor diet,

It's as simple as this. My facial firming program will help prevent wrinkles, lines and sags well into your 60's, 70's and 80's. This is not a mere promise.

you'll obviously have to work harder to accomplish this goal. However, no matter what shape your face is in today, my firming routine will give your skin better tone and circulation and will improve your appearance.

You can even lose those double chins, and reduce the fine lines and wrinkles.

It's as simple as this. If you follow my facial firming program consistently, you will help prevent wrinkles, lines, and sags well into your 60's, 70's and 80's. This is not a mere promise. I have seen the living proof in older models I work with in the beauty business.

So, beginning today, while your friends are squandering their savings for face-lifts, you can smile, look better than they do, and still bank your money.

Facial Beauty Basics

Before we get into the actual firming routine, here are a few basic rules to make beauty a never-ending part of your life.

1. *Always wear sunglasses in sunlight.* The brightness will make you squint, which makes the muscles around your eyes and forehead form wrinkles that get deeper and unerasable as time passes. Some overcast days can be so bright that sunglasses are necessary. When there is snow on the ground, remember that the reflection of light from it causes you to squint and frown,

even if you can't see the sun. The skin around the eyes is very fragile, so protect it from the elements.

2. *Don't smoke or suck on pencils.* If you purse your lips continually, you will create wrinkles all around your mouth. Every time you puff on a cigarette, you are putting permanent lines around your mouth that will become very obvious when your lipstick bleeds into the furrows.

Yes, you can erase a good many of these lines. But why keep putting them in every day at the same time you're trying to take them out. Become aware of any habits you have that encourage wrinkles and frown lines. Only then can you start on the path to reversing them.

3. *Wear a mouthguard when you sleep.* I have discovered that this helps my face tremendously in many ways. It prevents me from clenching my jaw, grinding my teeth and pursing my lips. It also prevents me from snoring!

If you are under stress, you can do more damage to your lip and chin lines when you sleep than if you smoked four packs of cigarettes a day.

Grinding your teeth while sleeping creates many problems that are expensive to correct, such as:

- Your teeth become shorter and your jaw collapses. Correction: rebuilding your teeth with crowns to open your bite.
- Your teeth move, causing spaces and an unbalanced bite. Correction: braces and more grinding by the dentist to balance your bite.
- TMJ problems and headaches. Correction: medication and more dental work.

I first found out about the mouthguard when my son was on his high school football team and was told to get a mouthguard to protect his teeth while playing contact sports. I went to a sports store and purchased a mouthguard for $1.25. Following directions on the package, I created a custom-fit shield for his teeth.

A light went on in my head! Instead of spending a fortune at the dental office for a custom-made mouthguard, why not try this for my purposes? I couldn't quite believe it when I first tested it, but in just a few days I had proof that it really worked! Not only did the wrinkles in my lipline soften to the point of disappearing, but I now wake up every morning without the sore muscles of nighttime facial stress or my usual headaches.

4. *Try not to frown or squint.* Many people (including me) frown when they talk, think, or find themselves in a bright light. This causes permanent furrows and wrinkles in your forehead, especially between your eyebrows and around your eyes.

I broke this habit (in the privacy of my home) by wearing scotch tape on those areas. Once the tape was on, every time I unconcsciously frowned or squinted, I was stopped by the pulling and pinching of the tape. This made me instantly aware of how often and when I was engaging those muscles. Best of all, it helped me to express myself without the aid of facial grimaces.

After a few weeks, my face was so sensitized by the tape that I could even feel these muscles frown when I was out in public, without the tape. I had actually taken this unconscious habit, and made it conscious. Therefore, I could block it 24-hours a day. (Yes, I firmly believe that I do not frown in my sleep anymore.)

As time passed, I hit upon the idea of thinking pleasant thoughts and letting my face relax and smile. Not only did the furrows and wrinkles stop growing deeper, but they also started to fade. I was smiling much more frequently. I was happier and the people around me were happier.

5. *Keep your hands away from your face.* Leaning on your hands will cause wrinkling and stretching of your skin. It also damages your tender facial skin. There are many germs on your hands which can cause blemishes or a rash on your face. Wash your hands thoroughly before you touch your face to wash it, apply makeup or give yourself a beauty treatment.

6. *Sleep on a flat or small pillow, or a neck roll.* Sleeping on a large pillow can cause wrinkling and stretching of your facial skin. It can also tilt your head forward, which will encourage a double chin and wrinkles in your neck.

Have you ever awakened with creases or marks on the side of your face from squishing it during sleep? You can check this easily: just go to your mirror immediately upon awakening. See if there are any creases or marks on the side of your face. Or has your chin multiplied overnight? Has your neck developed wrinkles across the front because your chin was resting on your chest?

All this can at least be partially prevented by using a neck roll or small pillow. They can support your neck perfectly and are small enough to maneuver when you change positions, so you will avoid the assault on your delicate facial and neck skin.

7. *Protect and support your neck.* One of the best discoveries I have made to prevent chin and neck aging is a soft cervical collar. Because of my headaches and mild cervical osteoarthritis, my doctor prescribed the soft collar to be worn while sleeping. He told me that, while I sleep, I get into positions that strain and cramp my neck muscles. Those positions also misalign the neck vertebrae, causing painful pinching of the nerves.

All this was true, but what he never thought about were the additional effects of these positions in creating double chins and facial and neck wrinkles. Now, by sleeping with this cervical collar, I have not only eliminated my awakening with a headache and a "charley horse," but I also found that my double chin and the wrinkles in my neck were disappearing.

Try
to be
aware
of slight,
sudden
movements
in your
face
so you
can stop
them
before
they
make
permanent
wrinkles.

8. Avoid facial twitches. Nerves play tricks on you, and most of the time show up in the form of facial twitches or "tics." Usually, you are not aware of them so ask a close friend to keep an eye on you for a while and tell you what twitches you have when you are deep in thought, or nervous. Try to be aware of these slight, sudden movements in your face so you can stop them before they make permanent wrinkles and lines. Besides, they are dead giveaways to your vulnerability and give the impression of a lack of composure or self-esteem.

Again, relax and let a little smile come across your face. Take a few minutes every few hours to "disappear" on a 60-second vacation into a beautiful beach scene, or with your children having fun, or making love, or any other imaginary adventure that relaxes and enthralls you. Above all, try to relax 6 times a day, at the very least.

You will find that, the more you do this, the less the facial twitches take over. And the vulnerability they reveal, the lack of composure or self-esteem that they exhibit to the world, will also pass out of your life.

Gentle Exercises To Firm Up
Your Face, Chin and Neck

NOTE: Controlling facial muscles is a slow, gradual process. Therefore, don't get discouraged if you do not see immediate results. It could take a month or two, but your efforts will be realized.

The first time you look into your mirror and see that your double chin has disappeared, you will realize how well-spent your time has been. No matter what shape your face is in today, you can lose those double chins.

Very Important Rules To Follow:

When massaging or applying creams to your face, always move your fingers *up* and to the *outside* of your face. When applying creams or foundation to the skin under your eyes, gently move your fingers from the *outside* of your eye to your nose.

Always cleanse your face and neck before you massage it. Use cream or oil so your fingers can move freely over your skin.

Do the following exercises once every day — preferably just after cleansing your face and neck.

Forehead and Furrow Between the Eyebrows

❖ Exercise 1

- Using the fingertips of your hands, massage the area between your eyebrows, alternating your hands.

- Move your left fingers up and out.

- Then, move your right fingers up and out.

- Repeat this move- ment 25 times.

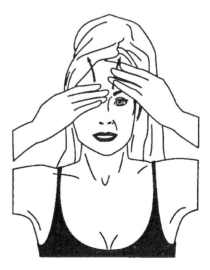

❖ Exercise 2

- Using the fingertips of your hands, start between your eyebrows and massage your forehead up and out to the sides.

- Left hand goes to the left.

- Right hand goes to the right.

- Repeat this movement 25 times.

❖ Exercise 3

- Place your left fingers on your left temple.

- Place your right fingers on your right temple.

- Make circles up and out.

- Repeat this movement 25 times.

These are good relaxers to be done throughout the day.

Eyelids and Crow's-feet

❖ Exercise 1

- Place your left fingertips at the outer corner of your left eye.

- Place your right fingertips at the outer corner of your right eye.

- Now, gently make circles up and out toward your ears.

- Repeat this movement 10 times.

❖ **Exercise 2**

- Massage your eye sockets in circles as follows —

- Place your fingertips at the inside corner of each eye.

- Gently move them from the nose, across the upper eyelid to the outer side of the eye, cross under the eye to the nose.

- Repeat this circle gently around each eye 10 times.

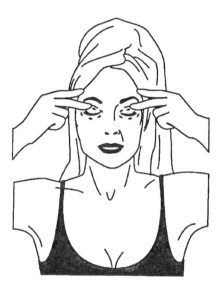

❖ **Exercise 3**

- Close your eyelids.

- Now try to open them without actually parting the lids.

- Try harder. (Feel the muscles trying to pull the eyelids apart, but don't let them.)

- Repeat 10 times.

This creates isometric tension on the muscles of your upper and lower eyelids and firms them up.

❖ Exercise 4

• Place your fingertips on each side of your nose.

• Gently pat the muscles across the top of your cheek-bones until you reach your temple.

• Repeat 10 times.

❖ Exercise 5

• This exercise is done with your eyes alone.

• First stare straight ahead.

• Then make a circle with your eyes looking as far as possible to the north. Then to the east. Then to the south. Then to the west. Then to the north.

• Repeat this circle 5 times to the left. Return your eyes to straight ahead. Close them and relax.

REVERSE

• Make the circles with your eyes rotating to the right 5 times.

• Return your eyes to straight ahead. Close them and relax.

Cheeks And Sides Of Your Face

❖ Exercise 1

• Place one finger vertically on both of your closed lips to prevent them from pursing.

• Relax your lips and keep them closed.

• Without opening or pursing your lips, blow your cheeks out.

• Look into the mirror to see your cheeks puffing out.

- Count to 5 and relax.

- Repeat 10 times.

This will help eliminate the line from the side of your nose to the corner of your mouth. It will also help eliminate those ugly little lines around your upper and lower lips.

❖ **Exercise 2**

- Smile broadly without parting your lips.

- Tense your cheek muscles as hard as you can, but do not let your lips part.

- Hold for a count of 10.

- Relax. Repeat 10 times.

This strengthens the "uplift" muscles in your cheeks and smoothes the wrinkles around your mouth.

❖ **Exercise 3**

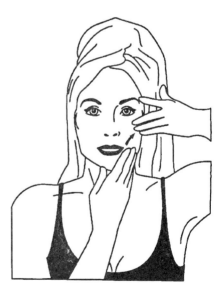

- Alternating your hands, use your fingers to massage up and out in the hollows of your cheekbones, from the corner of your mouth to your ear.
- Lift and smooth out the skin toward your ears.
- Go one way *only*. Always from mouth to ear. *Never* from ear to mouth.
- Repeat 10 times.

Tighten The Muscles Around Your Mouth

❖ Exercise 1

- Open your mouth as wide as you can.

- Curl your lips over your teeth. (This is essential. It is the curling over your lips that gives you the maximum effect.)

- Hold to a count of 5. Relax.

- Repeat 5 times.

❖ Exercise 2

- Place your middle fingers at the outside corners of your mouth. With small circular movements, massage your lips toward the top center.

- Then massage your lips back to the outer corners and proceed across the bottom lips toward the center.

- Massage your lips back to the outer corners.

- Repeat this sequence 5 times.

This will bring the circulation to your gums, teeth and lips. You will see your lips become fuller and more youthful.

Double Chin and Loose Neck Skin

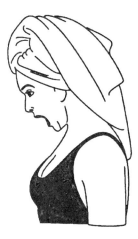

❖ Exercise 1

- Lower your chin to your chest.

- Open your mouth as wide as it will go.

- Raise your head and move it back as far as possible.

- Close your mouth tightly. (Feel your neck muscles stretch.)

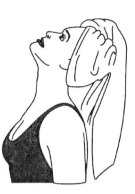

- Hold for a count of 10. Relax.

- Repeat 10 times.

❖ **Exercise 2**
- Open your mouth as wide as possible.

- Stretch out your tongue as far as possible.

- Hold for a count of 10. Relax.

- Repeat 10 times.

❖ **Exercise 3**
- Try to touch your nose with your lower lip.

- Hold for a count of 10. Relax.

- Repeat 10 times.

❖ **Exercise 4**
- Try to touch your nose with your tongue.

- Hold for a count of 10. Relax.

- Repeat 10 times.

Of course, you won't be able to make it, but the stretches will pull out the wrinkles in your neck.

❖ **Exercise 5**

- With your fingertips, smooth the skin under your jawbone from your chin to your ears. Go *only* from your chin to your ears. *Never* from your ears to your to your chin.

- Repeat 10 times.

❖ **Exercise 6**

- Let your head hang toward your right shoulder.

- Then let it drop to your chest.

- Roll it towards your left shoulder.

- Roll it towards the back, point your chin up.

- Return your head to an upright position.

- Repeat this movement 5 times to the left.

- Relax.

Then reverse and do this movement 5 times to the right.

❖ **Exercise 7**

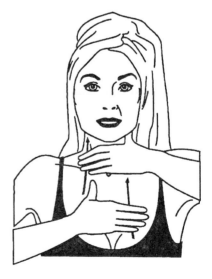

- Alternating your hands, use your fingers to massage your neck from your chest to your chin. Right hand goes up the left side, left hand goes up the right side.

- Move your hands only in an *up* and *out* direction.

- Repeat 10 times with each hand.

❖ **Exercise 8**

- To finish your routine, lie on your back with your head lower than your body. (Lie on your bed with your head hanging over the side.) Relax for 3 to 5 minutes.

This will bring the blood to your head for nourishment and to improve your circulation.

Carrying Your Head Gracefully

In order to carry your head with graceful mobility, you must have strong neck muscles. These isometric exercises will do the job.

❖ **Exercise 1**

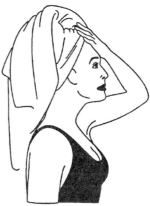

- Place the palm of your hand on your forehead and push.
- Hold your head steady as you resist the force of your hand.
- Hold for a count of 10. Relax.

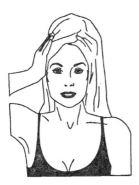

❖ **Exercise 2**

- Place the palm of your hand on the right side of your head above your ear and push.
- Hold your head steady as you resist the force of your hand.
- Hold for a count of 10. Relax.

❖ Exercise 3

  • Place the palm of your hand on the left side of your head above your ear and push.

  • Hold your head steady as you resist the force of your hand.

  • Hold for a count of 10. Relax.

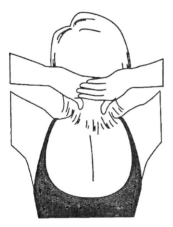

❖ Exercise 4

  • Place both hands behind your head and push.

  • Hold your head steady as you resist the force of your hands.

  • Hold for a count of 10. Relax.

Repeat all the above neck isometrics in sequence 5 times.

Gentle, Gentle, Gentle

When you do any of my exercises, you must concentrate on moving smoothly and gently. This is absolutely essential with your face. These facial exercises are meant to be effortless.

Remember, you want to firm the skin of your face — not stretch it. Therefore, treat it as though you were touching the face of a beloved child. When you massage it, massage it with love.

As with your body, you *coax* your face into firmness. This is why I believe that no plastic surgeon's knife can ever give me the results I've gotten from these gentle exercises. Remember, exercise restores the elasticity and firmness that you have lost over the years.

The skin of your face, as well as the skin of your body, has one amazing, forgotten capability! Top models use it to look young at seventy.

Your skin will automatically fit around whatever lies under it. If your muscles are stretched or sagging, your skin will stretch and sag with them. But, if your muscles become taut and firm, then your skin will shrink back to the same firmness.

A good example is when you are pregnant. Your abdomen expands with the growth of the baby inside it. After the baby is born, the abdomen muscles will shrink and return to the pre-pregnancy state *if you exercise* those muscles to firm them again. Notice how the skin shrinks along with the toning of your muscles.

STEP TWO: SKIN CARE

One of the first and most obvious places that aging shows up is in your face, neck and the back of your hands. You will see wrinkles, dry skin, sagging skin, and a sallow color.

The skin is your largest organ. It is a living organ that breathes. It allows the release of toxic wastes from the body in the form of perspiration. That perspiration also acts as a cooling system. *So your skin must be kept clean and supple.*

Your skin allows the oils of the glands under the skin to rise to the surface and lubricate the cells. The circulation in your blood vessels brings nourishment to your skin which gives it the healthy glow and color of youth. *So your circulation must be able to flow freely.*

The cells of the skin have a short lifespan. When they die, they must be sloughed off to make room for the new cells. This happens quite naturally when you are young. *So your skin must be kept moist.*

With these methods, and because the skin is a living membrane, you can reverse the signs of aging very easily.

My Daily Skin Care Program
For Face, Neck And Hands

The following applies to normal or dry skin.

1. Wash your face and neck with a gentle face cleanser. (I prefer only the type that can be removed with water.) Use a terry washcloth to gently rub the surface dirt and dead cells away.

2. Rinse thoroughly with lukewarm water. Pat dry with a towel.

3. Moving your fingers in an up and out direction, apply a non-alcoholic face toner to your face, eye area and neck. This will remove any residue and balance the PH in your skin. Do not use a toner with alcohol unless you have oily skin. The alcohol robs your skin of oils. I use Lancôme's *Tonique Doucuer*, but there are many other good toners on the market. You can try different brands to see what works best for you.

4. Moving your fingers in an up and out direction, apply a skin nourishing treatment to your face and neck. (Do not apply in the eye area.) I use Elizabeth Arden's *Ceramide Time Capsules*. Here, again, there are many companies that put out good facial treatments. Try different ones until you find one that makes your skin look alive.

5. After 5 minutes, apply a daytime moisturizer to your face and neck, moving your fingers in an up and out direction. (Do not apply to the eye area.) I use different moisturizers depending on the dryness of my skin on a given day.

When the weather is dry, I find my skin needs a heavier cream, sometimes even a night cream. On a warm, moist day, I use a light moisturizer.

Your skin should feel moist and supple to the touch. This is important for creating a smooth surface that your foundation can glide over easily without sinking into your pores.

6. *The eyes*: The skin around the eyes is very delicate. It needs products that are made specifically for that area. The skin is so fine and thin that it is not able to support a cream meant for your face. It will pull your skin down into folds or wrinkles. The heavier creams also migrate into the eyes and can irritate them.

If you have puffy lids, there are a number of remedies. Cool wet tea bags will take the puffiness out. Place one over each eye, lean back and rest for 5 minutes. Slices of cucumbers or potatoes will also do the job. The best prevention is to cut back on the salt in your diet. Water retention shows up immediately in droopy folds of skin in your upper eyelids.

There are good gels and creams on the market that have been proven to work wonders for puffy eyes and dark circles. My favorite is *Eye Contour Gel* by Clarins. When applying anything around the eyes, do not go all the way to the lashes because you risk getting it into your eyes.

Wait for 10 minutes so the gel can do its work. Then apply an eye cream to soften the fine wrinkles around the eyes. I follow the gel with *Eye Contour Balm* by Clarins. When my eye area is especially dry, I use Lancôme's *Progrès Eye Cream*.

7. Don't forget your lips. They need moisturizers too. Particularly if you are a lip licker like me. I use *Lip-Fix Crème* by Elizabeth Arden. I find it softens the lines around my lips and holds my lip liner in place. Throughout the day, I reapply *Lip-Fix* or *Carmex* to keep the softness on my lips.

Now I am ready to apply my makeup (*See* Step Three).

Here are some additional skin care treatments that should be done periodically. Almost every cosmetic and skin care company has a product for each treatment. Be sure to specify your skin type when you shop. A good way to test these products is to get the gift with purchase that each company has during their sales promotions. Or you can ask for samples. The companies I have found to be consistently above average are Lancôme, Clarins, Clinique, Elizabeth Arden and Estée Lauder.

1. *Dead Skin Removal:* the product for this is usually referred to as a polishing cream, a sloughing cream, or an exfoliating cream. I prefer a cream that has very tiny granules. This type is easier on your skin and leaves you with a fresh, clean glow. I equate it to the polish Tiffany would use on their silver.

Once a week, after removing your makeup, apply this cream to your wet face and neck. Do not touch the eye socket area. Massage gently with a terry washcloth or sponge. Always work in circles that go up and out. Be careful not to rub too hard or too long. Your skin is delicate — treat it like a fine piece of porcelain. Rinse well with warm water and pat dry with a towel.

2. *Deep Pore Cleansing, Nourishing, and Skin Tightening Mask*: The best time to get the most benefits from this treatment is right after you have completed the Dead Skin Removal treatment. Each company has the directions printed on their product. Follow them.

Once a week, after you have polished your face and neck, apply the mask gel, cream or mud to your face and neck. *Avoid the eye area and lips*. Lie down and rest for 10 minutes. I like to put cool tea bags, or cotton pads dipped in cold face tonic, over my eyes. Then rinse off with warm water and a washcloth or sponge (some masks have to be peeled off). Do this slowly and gently to avoid stretching the skin.

Then follow the daily routine, starting with your face tonic.

STEP THREE: MAKEUP TO ENHANCE YOUR BEAUTY

What does it do for you? Makeup can enhance the good features of your face. It can also conceal or underplay the features you want to improve. A rule of the art of makeup is: light shades make an area stand out, dark shades make an area recede or disappear in the overall picture.

The most important thing to remember about applying makeup is that it should not show. You must blend the edges of each shade you use into the surrounding area. This will create the illusion that all the colors and shadings you have used are really your natural beauty shining through.

It will eliminate forever someone looking at you and thinking, "Why does she wear so much makeup?" Instead they will say, "What beautiful eyes you have," or "How young you look today."

Even makeup artists will apply a lot of makeup, but when they are finished, you'd swear that face had almost no makeup on. *The secret is in the blending. There are no lines that stop with one shade and start with another.*

Think of yourself as an artist as you look into your mirror. Your face is the palette that you are going to paint a beautiful picture on, to bring out the beauty of your eyes and lips, and the rest of your face.

You will shape your face with shadings and color. A general rule in applying shadings is to go a shade lighter if you want to lift the dark areas or make them stand out. Go a shade darker if you want to make something recede or seem to disappear.

Now Let's Begin My 10-Minute Model's Makeup Routine

1. Apply a foundation that is the same tone as your skin color. It will create a clean palette for your accents. Cover your whole face and eye area with a thin coating. If you are wearing a low cut neckline, you may want to include your neck,

down to the place where your blouse or dress starts. This will camouflage freckles, sun damage and age spots. Blend it evenly all over so you cannot tell where it starts or ends.

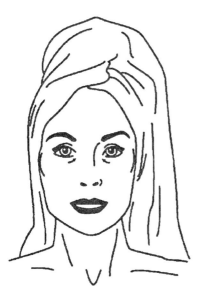

2. Most people have dark circles under their eyes. If you do, use an under-eye concealer that is a shade lighter than your foundation. Pat the concealer lightly *only* on the dark area under your eyes. If you have puffy eyes, do not put under-eye concealer on the puffy area. That will only emphasize the puffiness.

Remember, your skin is thin and delicate. Do not drag your fingers or you will stretch the skin and create wrinkles.

A tip: When you apply cream or makeup around the eyes, it is important to do it from the outside of your eye towards your nose.

And be sure to blend the edges into your foundation so you can't tell where one shade begins and another shade ends.

3. Next is the area from the eyebrow to the eye bone (the boney ridge where your eyelid starts). To be more specific, hold a pencil or ruler from the outer corner of your nostril to the outer corner of your eye opening. Draw an imaginary line from the corner of your eye to your eyebrow. Where that straight measure ends is where your eyebrow should end. This will give you the line bordering the outside of your upper eye area that is to be shadowed.

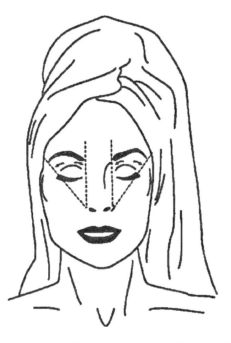

Apply a soft shade of rouge, eye shadow or shading to the area from your eye bone to your eyebrows. Cover the whole area, from the curve of your nose to the imaginary line on the outside of your eye.

If you have brown, black or red hair and your skin tone has a lot of beige or yellow in it, use a color that looks like soft clay, umber, ginger or any earthy shade with a brownish-peach tint. If you have white, silver or blonde hair with a pale skintone, use a shade that is a soft brownish-pink.

4. Your upper eyelid is a muscle that extends from your eye bone to your lashes. Here is where the folds and wrinkles show up. Be sure it is well-lubricated with an eye moisturizer that won't slide into the eyes. You can use a product called *Eye-Fix* by Elizabeth Arden. This will help your eye shadow stay put.

If you have deep-set eyes, use a powder or cream eye shadow that is light in color. Again, be sure not to lay it on heavy. It will only weigh down your delicate skin, creating more folds and wrinkles.

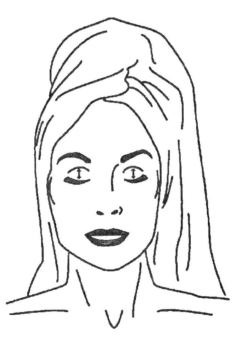

Frosted eyeshadows and colors such as blue, green and white are harsh and outdated. They are very unflattering and emphasize the wrinkles and folds. Stick to the soft matte neutrals. Beige, pale gold, peach, apricot, pale pink, and light lavender are colors that will go with everything and look natural.

Apply the eye shadow to your eyelid, from the eyelashes to the eye bone — from your nose to the imaginary line at the outer corner of your eye.

5. The Shading: Using a brush or sponge, shade under the eye bone to create the illusion of deep set eyes. Use an earthy tone such as, a medium brown, a light grey, or a midnight purple. This has to be blended so well, up and out, into the area above the eye bone that it appears to be a shadow.

With a brush and a light or medium brown shadow, lightly shade *under* the cheekbone to emphasize that cheekbone and create a hollow. The shadow should start directly under the cheekbone, about midway from your nose to your ear. Carry it through to your ear, following the underside of your cheekbone. It is most important that you blend this shading or else it will look out of place.

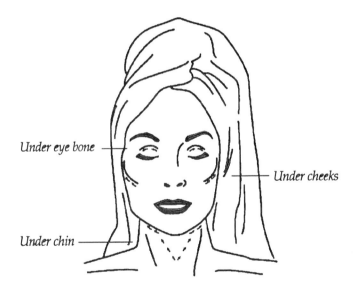

Under eye bone

Under cheeks

Under chin

The final shading is under your chin line to camouflage the loose skin or double chins. Using your shading brush and a light or medium brown shadow, follow under your chin bone and shade from one side to the other. This will give the illusion of a sharp chin line. Be sure to continue the shading across the double chin or chins, working into a V down the front of your neck.

Blend, blend, blend. The secret to successful camouflage!

6. The eyeliner is an option that can be used only if you soften it so it looks like an extension of your eyelids. There is nothing more harsh and artificial than to see a hard eyeliner on someone's eye. Unless, of course, you are doing theatrical makeup.

Use charcoal grey, midnight purple, or charcoal brown. These are colors that would appear naturally when you don't have makeup on. I prefer a soft pencil instead of a liquid eyeliner because it has an oil base that melts and can be softened with a Q-tip, brush or sponge on a stick. I find that my eyeliner melts within an hour and blends into the shadow of my eyelid. The color remains, but it is not a sharp, harsh line.

The whole idea of an eyeliner is to make your eyelashes appear longer and your eye opening appear to be larger.

7. Next comes your mascara. Black is standard. If it looks too harsh for your coloring, you can try charcoal brown or charcoal grey. Do not use blue, green or any other color except at night, or if you want a costume look.

The application is very important. Partially close your eyes and run the mascara wand across your lashes to color the tips (top and bottom). Use a lash brush or comb and separate them, removing the excess mascara. Apply a second coat with your eyelids open. Stroke from the roots toward the tips. If your lashes clump together, use a brush or comb to separate them.

8. A dusting of powder is next. This will set your makeup so it doesn't look greasy. It will also make it stay in place all day.

Do not use a tinted powder. Your foundation was selected to match your skin tone. If you use a tinted powder, you will end up with a darker shade on your face that will look artificial. I use a fine-grained, transparent loose powder and apply it with a big, fluffy brush. I find a cake powder leaves too much powder on my face. It emphasizes the wrinkles and looks heavy.

Lightly touch the brush on your powder. Tap the brush on the palm of your left hand until the powder remaining on the brush is just a light dusting. Now, moving it in small circles from the outside of your eye toward the nose, lightly take away the shine.

Then tap your brush on the palm of your hand to pick up some more powder and make sure your nose gets a good dusting. That's where most of the oil on your face will be produced throughout the day.

Next, picking up more powder from your hand, lightly brush over your cheeks and forward. Be sure to brush over your eye area from your eyelids to your eyebrows.

You will be amazed how a light dusting of powder will unify and blend the colors on your face, making it appear as if it had the natural beauty you were born with. And, it acts as a setting agent to hold your makeup in place all day.

9. The final touch: A little rouge to bring the glow of health to your palette. Everyone looks better with a rosy glow to their cheeks. For olive or yellow-tinted skins, use a peach, clay, or apricot shade. For ivory or pale skins, use a pink shade.

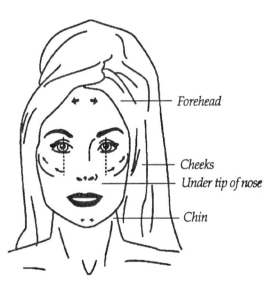

Forehead

Cheeks
Under tip of nose

Chin

With a fluffy brush, apply a light dusting of rouge on your cheeks from the center of your eye to the tip of your ear. Sometimes it helps to smile and apply the rouge to the tops of the cheeks.

A few tips to make your face look even younger and healthier. Brush a glow of rouge at the very top of your forehead — on the tip of your chin — and under the tip of your nose. When you think about where the sun colors your face, you will understand why color on these areas will make you glow with health.

10. The last touch of color is on your lips. Your eyes and your lips are the most memorable part of your face. Always keep a soothing balm on your lips to prevent dryness and cracking of the skin. My favorites are *Lip-Fix* by Elizabeth Arden and *Carmex*.

The general rule is to wear a color that compliments your skin tone. Earthy brownish-orange, apricot, or orange-red compliment redheads, brownettes and blondes with olive and yellow-tinted skin.

Pinks and reds with a blue base compliment blondes, brunettes, and grey or silver hair with fair skin.

Start with a lip liner pencil in the shade of the lipstick you plan to wear. Color in the edge of your lip line. Try to make the points at the top of your lips the same on both sides. Round the points to give a soft effect. It gives the impression you are tolerant and easy-going. Sharp points are harsh and make you look intolerant and inflexible. Draw the lines on the top lip all the way to the outer corners of your mouth.

Draw the lines on your bottom lip from the outer corners toward the center. Full, soft lips give a very youthful appearance. If you have thin lips, you can make them appear fuller by drawing the lip line just a touch outside of your natural lip line. Be sure to color it all the way to the natural lip line or it will look sloppy. Fill in your upper and lower lips with the pencil liner.

Then, apply your lipstick inside the outer line you have drawn. A trick to make your lips look fuller and more lush is to use a lighter shade over the top part of your lower lip.

There you have it — my 10-minute, 10-step makeup routine.

If you follow the three basic steps of my facial and neck beauty care program, I promise you will look younger and more beautiful.

And, most important of all, you will feel much younger!

24

Imaging — Who Is That Beauty?

What image do you project? What do people see when they look at you? Would you believe that *what they see influences how they perceive you to be*! First impressions are lasting impressions. They may not convey who you really are, but your outer image affects other people's opinions of you and how they relate to you.

You've heard the old adage, "Beauty is in the eye of the beholder." That's true! What vision are you presenting to the world? "But," you say, "true beauty comes from within, and is created by your spirituality and interactions with your fellow man." You're absolutely right! However, your inner beauty becomes evident over a period of time, as someone gets to know you. This chapter will deal with the more immediate visual outer image you present to the world — the way you package yourself.

Does your image say, "Hey, I love myself and life is wonderful," or "I'm moving up in this world," or "I may be over 40, but I have a lot more of life to live and I intend to enjoy every minute."

What the world sees is a reflection of what you feel about yourself and that message is sent by —

❖ The way you use clothes to create an attractive appearance.

❖ The way you take care of your skin.

Knowing how to put yourself together can take 10, maybe 15 years off your appearance. Enhancing your image is one of the easiest ways to give yourself an emotional and physical uplift.

❖ The way you use makeup — or not.

❖ Your hairstyling and color.

❖ The way you take care of your body.

❖ Your attitude in the way you move.

❖ And how you put it all together!

That's what I call "packaging" or "imaging."

Knowing how to put yourself together visually can take 10, maybe 15 years off your appearance. Enhancing your image is also one of the easiest ways to give yourself an emotional and physical uplift.

Try this little game during your next stroll down the street. Take a good look at a stranger and allow your thoughts to create a scenario of that person's character, self-esteem, age and lifestyle. You may be completely off base from the real truth! But you can bet that, without realizing it, you have determined what you believe that person to be based on what they are wearing, their hair and makeup, body size, body language, and how they have put it all together.

For instance: You see a woman approximately 45-50 years old — 20 lbs. overweight. She is wearing grey sneakers, blue socks, brown full skirt to mid-calf, brightly colored flowers on her cotton blouse (a little snug in the chest area), a grey baseball jacket with advertising on the back, no makeup to cover the dark circles under her eyes, and straggly hair with grey roots showing under faded brown. (Sounds a little extreme but I have seen images like that.)

What is your story of her lifestyle, her work, her feelings about herself, her attitude towards life, her personality, etc.? Be honest, you will never know her and no one will ever know what you are thinking. You can't help but have subconscious opinions that are not based on reality, but solely on visual impressions.

My visual impression is of a woman who thinks very little of herself — she has low self-esteem. Perhaps she never fulfilled her dreams, so became disillusioned with life. The way she dresses her body indicates no desire to look good. Her weight problem could be the result of eating to fill a void, or not feeling she is entitled to a good life. Perhaps she feels that no one cares, so why should she care. Her attitude is probably to just survive each day because there is nothing to look forward to. There is no joy in this picture, no zest for life. She looks older than she probably is.

That's just the imagery that comes to my mind when I see what that person presents to the world visually. I don't know her and probably will never run into her again. She may be completely different from my impression of her. How do you suppose that image would affect her encounters and relationships in life — her quality of life?

The same holds true for how you see yourself. I know that when I look at my image in the mirror, I feel different stages of like or dislike for who I appear to be which actually affect my mood and sense of well-being. When I am feeling low and vulnerable, I dress myself up, put on a little makeup, and fix my hair. Then I try to think positive: "I'm all right! I am strong! Things will get better! Have faith! This, too, shall pass!" My body language reflects these thoughts and I walk with confidence and a higher self-esteem. The transformation does wonders for me and is reflected in the responses I receive from others.

> One of the major factors in staying youthful and alive is sustaining a feeling of joy and hope — an excitement about what is going on — a contentment with who and where you are.

There Is Beauty in Everyone!

Although many cultures revere the mature woman and man, our culture has made *youth* the ideal. With a little awareness of how to enhance your beauty, you can very simply bring more zest into your life. Your psyche would love to be treated like a princess, so why not indulge yourself with a new look. In my 35 years of working in the world of beauty enhancement, I have learned many secrets. There are tricks of illusion (believe me, I have used many of them) and there are do's and don't's of good taste.

The predominant visual signs of aging are:

1. Sagging Breasts
2. Sagging Derrière
3. Wrinkles
4. Thinning Hair
5. Bulging Tummy
6. Flabby Arms
7. Cellulite
8. Chicken Neck
9. Double Chins
10. Sagging Jowls
11. Spider Veins
12. Age Spots
13. Sagging Eyelids
14. Greying Hair
15. Furrows in Lips
16. Dry & Aging Skin

Each one of these can be camouflaged to some extent and, in some cases, they can be completely corrected.

1. Sagging Breasts

Believe it or not, simple, quick chest exercises work! I have certainly proved that myself. Perseverance will pay off. But in the meantime, you must wear a good fitting bra for support and to prevent the further breakdown of your supporting muscles. The no-bra attitude is not for you.

2. Sagging Derrière

Here again, exercise does pay off! Until you have accomplished good muscle tone, a girdle will pull that flesh back up where it belongs.

3. Wrinkles

The talk of the nation! To have or not to have — has created anxiety in women — and men. Many say that wrinkles give a man's face character — and yet, wrinkles on a woman's face are considered undesirable. Here again, we are victims of our society's ideals — in a society where aging brings more respect, wrinkles are not considered a problem. If you consider wrinkles a problem, there are ways to deal with them. The most ideal method is to take care of your skin from your teenage years on and break any habits of frowning and squinting. That way you get a head start on preventing or prolonging the time that wrinkles will appear.

If you have already seen their formation and desire to minimize them, a good moisturizer is a necessity, to keep your skin moist at all times. There are also skin tightening creams, particularly for around the eyes, that do work. Try many different brands, from the inexpensive to expensive, to see what works best on your skin.

Everyone's skin is unique and will react differently to a product than someone else's. Your skin is a living organ that changes constantly, with new skin cells being formed and dead cells being sloughed off every day. That's why it's possible to heal it and undo any damage that has been created by bad nutrition, chemicals and the outside elements you are exposed to.

Wear sunglasses to prevent squinting and stress in the muscles around the eyes from bright lights. Refrain from frowning. I have put scotch tape on my forehead and bridge of the nose whenever I am alone, to make myself aware of the times I frown. But I wouldn't put tape around the eyes

The ideal method is to take care of your skin from your teenage years on and break any habits of frowning and squinting.

It's amazing how stress affects your whole body, particularly showing up in numerous wrinkles on your face.

because that skin is much too thin and sensitive. Exercise and massage can also minimize the wrinkles on your face and neck.

Try different types of stress relievers to help you relax. It's amazing how stress affects your whole body, particularly showing up in numerous wrinkles on your face.

If you don't have the patience to work with your skin, there is always cosmetic surgery and/or peeling to alter the course of your face. I personally hope the day never comes when I will feel that is my only alternative, because I feel that a part of my whole persona will change. I believe that one alteration leads to another, and another, and another, etc.

4. Thinning Hair

This can happen at any age. Although time and again, some new product shows up on the market that is supposed to create new hair, chances are that the hair follicle which ceases to produce will not be revived.

There are numerous products that will give your hair body, enable you to style it, and hold it in place. And wigs and hairpieces have done wonders for both men and women. Ask your hair stylist or a friend to show you how to use them.

But if you feel all the above is too much for you to deal with, you might want to try root transplants. Many have found that to be very successful.

5. Bulging Tummy

As you get older:

❖ Your metabolism slows down and so do your active activities.

- ❖ The fat that used to burn off will settle around your waist, stomach and hips.
- ❖ The lower activity level causes the muscles that support the abdomen and upper body to lose their tenacity.
- ❖ Gravity becomes the stronger force and your supportive muscles become like old rubber bands.

The spreading of your mid-section is a signal to reassess your nutritional intake, the only way every model I know has lost that mid-section spread. You need less food if you are operating on a lower activity level. You must also involve yourself in activities that will strengthen your muscles and build up your metabolic rate. Lose fat and tone your muscles for support! That is the only way to lose the mid-section spread.

Until your muscles can do a full-time job of supporting your abdomen and upper body, you will need help via a girdle. Liposuction and surgery are alternatives, but they do nothing for your muscle tone. Consequently, as time goes by, you will be back in the same dilemma.

6. Flabby Arms

Do your underarms wave when you raise your arms? Lack of muscle tone again! Muscles that are not used will atrophy and sag. These are so easy to smooth out with simple exercises done three times a week.

Until you tighten up, the only camouflage is sleeves that cover your upper arms.

7. Cellulite

"The little dimples that show up in your fatty areas." Yes, I certainly used to have cellulite. Once upon a time. Long ago. And you'll say the same. Spas and beauty products claim to be able to rub away your dimples, but the only way I was ever able to make them disappear was to lose weight to melt the fat away and tone up my muscles. And believe me, I have had to reassess and take action several times throughout my life.

8. Chicken Neck

Sounds so unattractive, but that is exactly what I'm reminded of when I see skin hanging like Austrian shades at the base of the neck. Add to that — dry, tough skin that has been damaged by the weather — and you have an undesirable effect of aging.

Prevention is your best ally. But, if your neck is already losing its swanlike appearance, there are a few remedies that can soften the effect.

Facial and neck exercises can tighten the foundation of the skin. Hold your head erect, lengthen the back of your neck, and relax your shoulders. This simple posture will strengthen the muscles of your neck and help prevent wrinkling.

Moisturizer at all times is a necessity. Your neck skin is just as fine and thin as the skin on your face. Most people pamper their face and forget that the neck is an extension of it. Camouflage or coverups include necklaces, scarfs, turtleneck and mock turtle necklines. Makeup will also even out the skin tone and camouflage any aging spots.

9. Double Chins

You can apply a shading rouge to minimize fullness.

Some people have more than one. Losing weight, facial and neck exercises have done the job for me in the past. Liposuction and surgery to get rid of double chins should be a last resort.

Under your chin, you can apply a shading rouge or a shade darker makeup than your face makeup to minimize the fullness there.

Here again, good posture can reduce double chins. When you constantly tuck your chin in by looking downward or letting your head hang, you create folds under your chin and wrinkles on your neck. So, sit tall, walk tall, hold your head erect and your whole body will feel stronger and lighter.

10. Sagging Jowls

I do believe I've found an instant remedy — smiling. It is one of the best ways to minimize those flaps that start to grow on the sides of your chin. Look into the mirror with a relaxed face. Now, smile and watch those little flaps blend into your jawbone. Isn't it wonderful how a smile can change your whole outlook?!

The shading rouge and the under-the-chin makeup will also sharpen your jawline.

Acupuncture is a possible remedy for sagging muscles. It has been noted to stimulate the facial muscles that can lift the downward pull of gravity.

Believe it or not — smiling is one of the best ways to minimize those flaps that start to grow on the sides of your chin.

11. Spider Veins and Varicose Veins

Two very different conditions. Spider veins are the tiny red veins that appear right under the skin. They look like country roads on a road map. These can be covered with your face make up, leg makeup, or the special makeup used for birthmarks and scars. Be sure to match the color of your skin. They can also be medically removed by your doctor.

Varicose veins are a bulging of the vein due to a weakness in the walls of the vein. You might try covering these with makeup if you consider them unsightly. However, they should be checked by your physician to determine if they need to be medically removed for your health's sake.

12. Age Spots

Those little, or large, brown spots that some people call "liver spots." These are usually harmless, flat discolorations that can easily be covered by makeup.

13. Sagging Eyelids

A dilemma that knows no age limits. They can be caused by a hangover, excess fluid in the body, mosquito bites and many years of gravity at work.

Ancient remedies include wet tea bags, cucumber slices, cornstarch paste, egg whites and ice packs. There are many products on the market, made specifically for the eye area, that will tighten the skin for a period of time. Be sure to use moisturizer around the eyes after these astringents do their work, or you will find the skin drying out and wrinkles showing up.

Makeup, shading and eyeshadow can be used to minimize the visual effect of excess skin.

My eyelids have started to sag dozens of times, but every time I "sucked the sag" out of them by backing off on my salt intake. Too much salt causes water retention in my body and shows up in my eyelids. You never have to use the salt shaker because there is salt in almost everything you eat, particularly in processed and canned foods, meats, soups, and every meal you eat in a restaurant.

For some people, surgery is necessary if their vision is impaired. Others have it for cosmetic reasons. I am in favor of trying everything possible before considering physical alterations.

14. Greying Hair

I have seen people with greying hair in their early twenties. It can happen at any age. Grey, silver, salt and pepper, and white hair are beautiful. Yet, they cast the illusion of aging or growing old.

If you don't want to flaunt your silver hair, *color it*! Yes, color does make you look younger. It gives more body to your hair and can liven up your skin tone. Try on different colored wigs to see what color does the most for your psyche and appearance. Then have a professional colorist give you that color. If you are handy with your haircare, have someone show you how to do your own coloring or try the shampoo-in products at your local store. Please read and follow instructions.

15. Furrows In Lips

Not such a problem for men, but women have to deal with lipstick bleeding into the furrows. They are now treatable — and preventable — at last. Moisturizer is very important to prevent dry, cracked lips and the furrows around their perimeter. There are products on the market made specifically for these problems. I use *Carmex* or *Blistex* lip balm for dry and chapped lips and, on the perimeter of my lips, *Lip-fix* works well to prevent lipstick bleeding and to soften the furrows.

Cover the lip line with foundation, then powder. Draw the outline of your lips with a lip pencil that matches the shade of lipstick you will use. The pencil color will not bleed as easily as your lipstick.

Remember, smoking and pursing your lips make the furrows deeper. Chemical peeling is available for those who feel the need to soften their lipline.

16. Dry and Aging Skin

This is a condition that can affect anyone at any age. But there are many ways to keep your skin smooth and youthful from the outside — body lotions, oils, creams, mud packs, massages to stimulate the oil glands, etc.

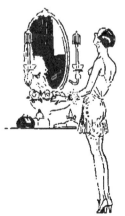

Good nutrition and vitamin supplements also contribute to the healthy function of your largest organ — your skin.

To sum up the above remedies for age prevention or reversal, it is obvious that *Activity, Exercise, Nutrition,* and *Attitude* are the major areas to which we must apply ourselves in order to live to the fullest capacity.

Now that I've covered the visual signs of aging, let's take a look at how to dress the body for a powerful and appealing impression.

A perfect figure (created by the advertising industry) is a rarity for 99% of humanity, young people included. The standard measurements formula starts with the bust — the waist should be 10 inches smaller, and the hips (7 inches below the waist) should measure 2 inches larger than the bust. Example:

❖ Bust 34

❖ Waist 24

❖ Hips 36

> There are ways to camouflage and balance a figure that does not have the above proportions to create the illusion of a more perfect figure.

Bodyshape

The bodyshape seems to fall into four categories —

❖ *Top heavy*: bust and upper arms larger than hips and thighs.

❖ *Bottom heavy*: hips and thighs larger than bust and arms.

❖ *Too big*: bulges and rolls.

❖ *Too skinny*: no shape, or few curves.

Let's get started. Stand nude in front of a full length mirror. Remember that you are perfect and unique in the eyes of your creator, no matter what shape you are in! Love and respect your body — that's where the real beauty begins. Now, having said that, decide which of the above shapes you resemble and what you want to camouflage for our culture, then make a list.

A great way to visualize what optical illusion can do for you is to study the windows of the large-size women's stores and the fashion magazines that are geared towards this category. Dress designers have come a long way in creating designs and lines that are flattering to the fuller figure. Study the way they layer clothing and the colors they use.

Below are some tips on how to create the illusion of what you would like the world to see.

Top Heavy

If you want to draw attention away from the top and focus on your pretty face or great legs, you can do it with the optical illusion of lines, colors and prints.

1. Necklines that expose cleavage will only draw attention to what you've got. Now this may be what you are looking for so be ready for those glances, comments and advances. If you shy away from such encounters, then wear a neckline that takes away from the obvious, such as a jewel neckline, mock turtleneck, boatneck, scoop neck or a blouse with a collar.

2. Wear colors that are soft or dark. Bright colors, bold prints and horizontal lines are killers, as they scream for attention and broaden the territory. If you like prints, be sure they are very small with little contrast.

3. Tight fitting sweaters or blouses will emphasize the size. Loose fitting sweaters or blouses will camouflage what's underneath. A jacket is a great equalizer. A suit with a touch of color from a pretty scarf at the neck will always flatter your figure.

4. Wear a bra that fits your size. When buying one, try a sweater over it to see if it creates bulges. A cup size that is too small will cause bulges and make you jiggle. You

If you want to draw attention away from the top and focus on your pretty face or great legs, you can do it with the optical illusion of lines, colors and prints.

also need good support. There are pretty bras with an underwire that will do the job and make you feel feminine. If you like to wear colored lingerie, be sure it doesn't show through your outer garment.

5. Heavy fabrics, stiff fabrics and bulky sweaters will make you appear bigger. Instead, wear soft fabrics such as silk, rayon, cashmere, rayon velvet, crepe, pima cotton, or batiste.

6. Sleeves that are slender, but not tight, will minimize your size. Stay away from raglan and batwing sleeves as they add more bulk to your top.

Bottom Heavy

If you want to draw the attention away from your hips and thighs, again, the optical illusions of lines, colors and prints are your tools.

1. Dark colors make you appear slimmer. Bright colors, bold prints and horizontal lines will call out, "Hey, look at me!" Use your prints and colors in blouses and scarfs.

2. Never wear gathers or pleats at the waist, you don't need the additional bulk. Empire waistlines are great for optical illusion, and skirts and slacks that fit the waist and taper down to a slim, A-line, or trumpet bottom will give you a flare with a slimming effect.

3. Jackets, vests and tunic tops can give a leaner line to the body, but be sure they cover your derrière. Mid-thigh and longer is a great length for these tops.

4. Heavy or bulky fabrics do not do justice to your waist, hips and thighs. Wear them on top to create a more balanced line. Soft, supple fabrics make skirts and slacks more graceful.

5. Wearing heels will give your body a longer, leaner look, but wear only what you can walk gracefully in. Four-inch heels may look great on models, but walking any distance can be disastrous. My feet ache at the thought of it, but even worse, think what your body language will be if you are in pain. A 2" heel is a good height for daytime and a 3" heel for evening or a special occasion, if you are not going to be on your feet for long.

Too Big

Big is Beautiful! You can enhance your image with classic styles. They usually have simple lines that are very flattering to anyone's figure. That's why they never go out of style.

1. Fabrics should be soft and supple — not clinging. For instance: fine wools, gabardine, rayon velvet, cotton. A fabric that has body to it so it doesn't hug the curves, yet soft enough to flow over them.

2. Neutral colors such as shades of grey, black, beige, brown, navy and maroon are wonderful for a head-to-toe cover. They minimize size. Bring your colors in through accents like scarfs, jewelry, a blouse with a suit, etc. Don't be afraid to wear bright colors and prints in your accessories. The splashes of color will lift your spirits and send the message that you enjoy life.

3. Undergarments are very helpful in shaping a large-sized body. I have found that properly fitted undergarments (with the help of someone who knows how to fit them) will not only enhance my figure, but have also made it more comfortable to carry around my excess weight.

Too Skinny

In our world of fashion, the skinny (or thin) body is desirable because it allows any fabric or design to be shown at its best, with no need to consider camouflaging a figure problem. However, the advertising world will play up the figure that has more curves. What is a woman supposed to do?!

If you fall into the "too skinny" category, consider yourself blessed. You can wear anything you desire. Bulky fabrics, bold prints, layers of clothing, stripes in any direction, etc. You can have a great time with any fashion design.

However, if you want to create the illusion of more curves, try the following:

1. For a fuller bustline, try a padded bra or stuff your bra with stockings (fleshtone, or match the color of your bra).

2. Bulky fabrics, sweaters, padded shoulders, layering, such as a cardigan sweater over another sweater, jacket over vest over blouse or sweater, etc., will add width to your top and camouflage a small bustline.

3. Pleated or gathered skirts add fullness to the hips. You can wear all the fun skirts — long or calf-length — that have a flare.

4. Wear slacks with full legs rather than the skinny stretch pants that call attention to thin legs.

5. Bathing suits can be your ally if you choose bright colors, bold prints or padded tops. Skinny hips look great in a bikini with a little ruffle.

There you have it! The top-heavy look is gone. The bottom-heavy look is gone. The too-skinny look is gone. The more-curves look is now yours instantly with these guidelines to help you improve your quality of life. They have worked for me and I hope you can benefit from my experience.

These guidelines can help you improve your quality of life. They have worked for me and I hope you can benefit from my experience.

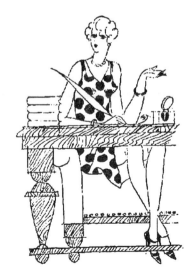

25

Mind, Body, Emotions, and Spirit

$\mathcal{I}$ n this age of awareness, a new phrase has been adopted: *Mind, Body, Emotions and Spirit*. What does it mean? Why and how are they linked together? Each of these components is a powerful entity within itself and its functions are described below, but the real power of life is evident when all four are functioning at peak performance, in sync with each other. Somewhat like the spark plugs of a car, when they are out of sync the quality of your ride leaves a lot to be desired. A vital, healthy, youthful, and enjoyable life is dependent on the full force of these four components working together in harmony.

Now let's see why each is important and you will realize how detrimental each can be to the harmony in your life.

Mind

Your mind is the Engineer, the Control Center of your body. It gives the commands for every movement of your body, whether it is voluntary or involuntary.

The voluntary moves are dictated by your conscious mind using the information you have programmed it with through your education, environment and life experiences from birth. You use this information to motivate your body into action

375

Nourish your mind's health with good nutrition, stress control, information gathering and positive thoughts.

and to make decisions about how you conduct your life.

The involuntary moves are programmed by a Higher Force and your subconscious mind. These are the movements that give you life and keep you alive, such as breathing, the functions of your organs, the constant rebuilding of your cells, the circulation of the fluids in your body and the protective responses to life's threatening stimuli.

Your mind is also the Library of your knowledge. It is the storehouse of all the information you have gathered along your path of life. Many people believe that you bring knowledge with you from previous lives, which might explain why some people have wisdom beyond their age. I'm sure you know or have heard of someone who has blown your mind with their in-depth knowledge of a subject that only a much older person would have had the time to accumulate. "That little boy sounds like such an old man," has been a statement I've heard so many times. We speak of the Gift of Talent that is present in outstanding artists. Perhaps it was a learned skill that was brought by the Life Spirit from a previous life or lives. It may have taken lifetimes of hard work to bring them to the present stage of accomplishment.

You have the innate capacity for creativity and achievement of your goals. However, you are on your own individual path and timespan so don't try to compare yourself to anyone else. Rejoice in your presence and carefully guard your mind's health. Nourish it with good nutrition, stress control, information gathering and positive thoughts. Without a healthy mind, your whole Being is adversely affected. In the chapter "Mind Power," you will learn ways to nourish and nurture your mind.

Body

The Temple — for your Soul, for the God within you, for your Spirit.

It is the vehicle for your Universal Being to travel on earth in this lifetime. Therefore, if you abuse it, you destroy your home. It is most vital to have a strong and healthy body if you are to have longevity in this lifetime, free from any illness that would interfere with the peak performance of your capacity for achievement and fulfillment of your desires.

Yes, it is possible for you to overcome the detriments of an unhealthy or afflicted body, but why add obstacles to your passage through life by neglect, when it is easier to maintain a healthy body that will assist you in all your endeavors. You are given a strong, flexible, miraculous body at birth and it is up to you to care for it and develop its strengths. (Admittedly, there are those who are born with what we have labeled "defects," but who is to say that these were not chosen by a Higher Being in order to develop more fully other attributes?)

I am speaking of the majority of humanity. Many people attribute my youthful appearance, agility and energy to heredity. Wrong! It is synergism (the theological doctrine that regeneration is effected by a combination of human will and divine grace). I know that my conscious efforts to strengthen and nourish my body from the time I was a young girl have prolonged its youthful vitality and slowed down its aging process. In Chapter 22, "Physical Fitness: Stretching and Exercising Give New Life!" and in Chapter 19, "Nutrition: The Key to Second Youth", you will find the ways that I have nurtured my body so it can assist me by performing at its peak.

Your body is an amazing vehicle in that it adapts so readily to rejuvenating efforts. That's why it is never too late to start caring for it and reversing the effects of your neglect. When you start to seriously consider your body as your Temple, your only Home on Earth, and you "clean house" or "shape up," you realize how important this vehicle is to your well-being and enjoyment of life.

Emotions

The Spice of Life! The Color of Living! To experience the full range of emotions — happiness/sadness, love/hate, empathy/apathy, reverence/obstinance, excitement/boredom, etc. — is to enjoy the Passion of living.

Without your emotions, you are no more than a robot. Your feelings are what make life interesting and give you the motivation to reach for higher goals. How can you enjoy the wonders of your world if you do not have emotions attached to what you see, hear and say? If you do not experience love, how can you relate to who you are in a positive way? If you do not experience sadness or boredom, how can you fully appreciate happiness, excitement or joy? No one likes to experience the negative emotions and yet they are the vehicles of transition in life.

If positive emotions were the only feelings you ever experienced, you would never be motivated to change your situation or circumstances. Imagine that you could feel only the positives . . . you are faced with the loss of your home because the rent was increased beyond your budget or the taxes went sky-high. You say, "I know everything will turn out right because I feel happy about living." Well, it won't. Unless you feel the emotions of fear and loss and anger, you will not feel motivated to alter the situation or change your circumstances. Or perhaps you are confronted by the loss of a loved one, but you do not feel the sadness of that loss. How can you know or recognize that love if you do not know the sad feeling of the loss of it? And how can you appreciate the feelings of another human being if you haven't experienced those emotions yourself?

Life's experiences would be empty without color and sensations. They educate us and create the physiological changes in our bodies which affect us and give us our perceptions of what we believe to be good or bad. This is what creates the Passion of Life.

Too often you grow up with defense mechanisms that obscure your true feelings and you become the image of what you think is acceptable for survival. In most cases, that image will rob you of the true happiness you are entitled to. You live the life that others have chosen for you and deny the real beauty of who you are. Be aware of your emotions and heed them. They are your teachers of what is really important in your individual life journey. Chapter 27, "Spirituality", will help you unlock the doors that have shut down your ability to live with real Passion.

Spirit

The God within you. The Light within you. Your Higher Self. Your Universal Soul. The Eternal Being that lives in your Temple on earth. Surely you have heard at least one of these phrases which describe the essence of creation within you. All of humanity is tied together with this thread of ethereal presence. It is the connection you have to all of mankind.

Be aware of your emotions and heed them. They are your teachers of what is really important in your individual life journey.

Spirit is where your inner strength and compassion comes from. You can see it at work when disasters hit, with people automatically banding together to help each other, without questioning race, color, religion, gender . . . all those categories used to divide us when we function within the framework of man-created society. Yes, there is a Higher Being within you that must be acknowledged and nurtured to complete the circle of your wholeness. Without the awareness of your spiritual core, you become an empty, shallow person. Your motivations become a dance of desperation to fill the void within and mask the discontent and emotional pain you feel.

When you are born, the Light within you is so evident in the free and open exploration of life. You delight in the search for new and exciting avenues to follow. As you grow and experience disappointment and criticism, that Light grows dimmer because of all the veils (or walls) you surround yourself with to protect you from the pain of the outer world called society.

But none of those protective devices are necessary if you learn how to trust and rely on your inner strength (your inner power) which has always been within you since your conception. Believe in yourself and know that all the answers you need to make your life what you want it to be lie within you. No one else can give you the answers that are right for your life.

When you nurture and trust that Light within, the glow of confidence, contentment and wisdom radiates from you and you are perceived as possessing the secrets of youth, happiness and power. How many times have you heard that someone has an aura about them or that they have charisma. They are in touch with their Spirit (or whatever you choose to call it), and have acknowledged it as the basis of their existence. Everyone has this Light within, but too many have lost contact with it. Life on earth is difficult! No one can argue with that. But when you learn to rely on your strengths from within and learn what tools are necessary to deal with the obstacles you encounter, there is no end to the successes you can bring about. The miracles of your life lie within you.

In the chapter on "Spirituality," you will find ways to get back in touch with your Inner Light, the real strength of your Being.

26

Meditation: The World's Easiest Way To Meditate

For four thousand years, there has been a simple, incredibly powerful tool to relax your entire mind, body and soul. It is called meditation, and it was known by the ancient Jews, Christians, Buddhists, Hindus and dozens of other communities.

Each community seemed to have invented its own path for reaching this deep healing tranquility. For penetrating into the inner space of their existence, and placing themselves a million miles away from this planet of stress, frustration and disappointment.

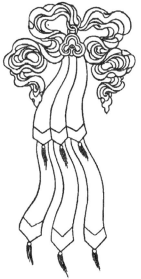

However, our Western civilization seems to have forgotten the value of this self-induced peace. We seem to prefer unending strife. We are therefore far too cruel to ourselves, and as a result we break down too quickly and too easily.

So we have attempted to learn from the Buddhists . . . the Yogis . . . the Cabalists . . . and the other mystics of every sort and persuasion. And many have succeeded in walking their paths.

But many others — perhaps you yourself — have found these paths unwalkable. Somehow, you can't reach your center that way. So perhaps you, like I for so many years, have given up that door to a higher existence. But now I have found the world's easiest way to meditate that works, almost from the very first time, takes absolutely no preparation, and combines youthful exercises with blissful escape.

Losing Yourself While Walking

Call it, if you will, losing yourself while walking. It begins, of course, by taking a 10 or a 15 minute pleasant walk. Not speed walking, just a relaxed stroll around the neighborhood of your home, or work, or wherever you find yourself at that minute.

To anyone who sees you, you will look like you're simply a person out walking.

Wear comfortable clothing, of course. Have a watch with you. Or, as I do, have an automatic timer that is set for half the time you want to walk.

For example, if you wish to walk for 10 minutes that day, set the timer for 5 minutes. Walk away from your home until the timer rings, then turn back and return to your house.

To anyone who sees you, you will look like you're simply a person out walking. But this vision of you will be deceptive because this time you are not going to focus on the familiar sights around you as you walk, but on your own breathing or the gently repeated feel of your feet as they touch the ground, one after the other.

Concentrate on that breathing as you walk. Or on those feet coming up and going down on that pavement. Hear nothing else. Pay attention to nothing else. Focus on nothing else.

Become your breath as you walk. Become the tread of your feet as you walk. Think of nothing for that 10 or 15 minute walk but that breath or the tread of those feet. Let every other thought slip gently out of your mind.

You are breath. You are movement. You are free.

Your mind loses its obsession with the world before or after that walk. It is isolated, shielded, liberated from that world. You are nothing more than your breathing in and breathing out and your feet moving forward one after the other. You are free. You are in another dimension. You are floating down that street, in the world but no longer of that world, with your soul being fed by the reality of your simplest possible acts . . . your breathing and your moving.

Once your mind is freed in this way, your body cannot help but respond. The body chemicals of worry, of stress, of tension, anxiety and fear all drain into your blood system where they can be worked out of your body by your movement.

You are the breath of life and the flow of movement. You are life and movement, and nothing more.

Before you know it you will be back at your starting point. It will be as though a

The body chemicals of worry, of stress, of tension, anxiety and fear all drain into your blood system where they can be worked out of your body by your movement.

minute, and a year, have passed. Time will have lost its meaning. Worry will have lost its power. And you will be ready to face life again, cleansed and renewed.

So easy, and yet so infinitely powerful. Why not take your first meditation walk . . . right now.

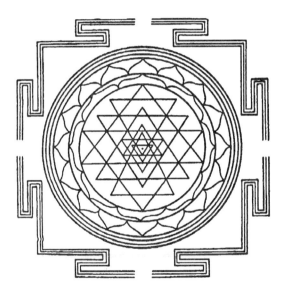

27

Spirituality

What is spirituality? It is an inner strength that supports and fortifies you in your daily journey down Life's path. It is a strong belief that there is a Higher Power which governs your life. Religions, cultures and philosophies are based on that belief.

I appreciate and respect all religions, cultures and philosophies. Each of them offers a source for education and gratification of the human spirit. Each person has reasons for following the religion of their choice and I believe that what works for you is the most important factor. As long as you have faith in the Higher Power, you have the opportunity to experience the true fulfillment of Life.

The more you understand the different philosophies, the more you will see that, even in the face of what you may conceive to be a tragic circumstance, there is a larger plan inside which your circumstance plays a part. Without an understanding of those sources, you would be tossed about like a ship without a rudder. A victim of unknown forces. So, faith in a Higher Power (whatever you believe it to be), is a source of solutions and comfort in the journey through everyday reality.

> The "Higher Power" is a common thread of Divine meta-physical energy that is present within all human beings, binding us together as brother and sister, regardless of race, color, creed or culture.

Some people believe that the Higher Power is outside themselves and give it a name such as God, Allah, Jehovah, Elohim, Yahweh, Vishnu, Brahma, Shiva, Buddha, etc., to whom they pray for guidance and protection. They see themselves as disciples of another being and, therefore, at their mercy. When a situation occurs, whether good or bad, they give the credit or responsibility to that outside power as though their own actions or desires are beyond their control. You may have heard — "God, why have you failed me," or "Thank you, God for coming to my aid," or "The devil made me do it."

Others believe that same Power to be within themselves as the "Higher Self," a plateau reached by spiritual self-awareness. They believe the "Higher Power" is a common thread of Divine metaphysical energy that is present within all human beings, binding us together as brother and sister, regardless of race, color, creed or culture.

Another reference to this "Higher Power" is "the God within you," or "the Divine in you." It is also known as "Your Intuition."

How Do I Get In Touch With My Higher Power?

Although your spirituality is innate, you must develop the skill of getting in touch with it through *knowledge* and *practice*. Just as in music, dance, writing, acting, sports, etc., fine-tuning comes with education and practice. There are many sources for gaining knowledge of philosophies that have been researched for centuries, and many self-help books and programs that have tried to simplify the steps to reach self-awareness.

The *telephone book* is a good source to start with. If you look up Catholic, you will find organizations that have classes, seminars, literature, audiotapes, videotapes, private counseling, retreats, etc. The same goes for Jewish, Muslim, Buddhist, Hindu, Zen, Yoga, or whatever spiritual or philisophical interest you have.

Churches, synagogues, temples, mosques, etc. are also very fruitful sources for material and practice. It is not necessary to be a member to enter, but be sure to respect their practices. Before you enter a place of worship that you are not familiar with, it would be advisable to ask if there are any practices you should follow, so you don't offend anyone. For instance, I have had to remove my shoes before entering a Mosque — on entering an Orthodox Synagogue, I had to place a covering on my head. Some places of worship have a restricted dress code.

I have studied and practiced different religions and philosophies throughout my life. Admittedly, my motivation was usually to escape the pain of my life's circumstances at the time. I have never considered spirituality a crutch (as some non-believers would call it), I see it rather as a positive search for tools to cope and deal with problematic issues, so I can experience the true joy of living.

Christianity, Catholicism, Judaism, Islam, Religious Science of the Mind, Zen (Buddhism), Yoga (Hinduism), etc., have their differences, but the common theme is that a Higher Power is Absolute — the Divine Truth. I have found that each time I lose sight of that Higher Power, my ability to cope with the everyday stresses becomes diffused and out of control. When I bring my spirituality into practice, my life takes on a whole new perspective and the problems I encounter are dealt with in a more productive way. The pain and pressure are lifted, and life becomes fun again. Stress, pain, pressure, denial — all are negative reactions that steal the bloom of our existence.

By gathering *knowledge* of the different philosophies that you have explored or will explore, you will develop your own beliefs in your spiritual awareness. You will also develop a greater understanding of why cultures differ. And yet, you will find that all human beings have the same basic emotions and sensitivities — that we are all Divine regardless of our differences.

The *practice* part comes through *meditation, prayer, mantras, chants, affirmations, actions, introspection, observation* and *analysis* of your past experiences, and a willingness to experience the unknown through faith. There are classes, seminars, books, and videos that teach you how to get the most value out of each form of practice. Believe it or not, there are short cuts and systems that will help you obtain the results you wish to achieve from your practice. And what a fascinating journey you will experience in seeking them out. I can guarantee that your life will take on a new perspective and move toward more fulfillment as you explore these new pathways.

Spirituality Is Different and More Powerful Than Just Having Positive Attitudes!

There are several components to realizing your spiritual power. Know that *Truth* is the Universal Power. What you see and believe is only your interpretation colored by your environment and past experiences. By not acknowledging your Higher Self, it is possible to become trapped in the "human experience." You believe that what you see and are experiencing is what must be accepted.

Spiritual realization is having *Faith*. Faith is an action of accepting that you are more than you appear to be and have a Higher Power that will guide you for the Goodness of Life.

Confidence comes from your understanding of who and what you are in relationship to the Universal Power, your Higher Self.

Healing is what transpires when you align yourself with the very essence of Life, your "Higher Self." Utilize the tools that are available to help you get out of the "human experience." Let the Power and Intelligence of your Life Force enable you to perceive a way to create an environment for yourself that opens the door to the new wonderful experiences of Life.

Who Am I? The Search for Self-Awareness

What makes a person beautiful? They may have a very pleasing outer appearance, but when you get to know them, they no longer seem beautiful. While another person, who may not have been as attractive at first, becomes more beautiful as you get to know them. Doesn't that tell you something about the inner quality of a person being the true beauty?

When you were born, you had complete self-awareness of your power. As you grew in your environment, your power was challenged and your beliefs were shaped by the world around you, many times negatively. Unless you lived in a spiritual atmosphere, you became indoctrinated by the human experience as a matter of emotional and physical survival. The older you got, the further you drifted from the true essence of your real self, creating, as a result, inner conflict, discontent and disillusionment with your life. And how can anyone be truly happy and enjoy life to the fullest under those circumstances? I have found my own quest for spiritual awareness and my true identity to be fascinating and liberating.

Self-esteem, contentment with yourself, positive acceptance of who you are, enjoyment of life, a true enjoyment of others. . . all these aspects of a person's inner life create an aura that is magnetic to others. They also enable you to go through the problematic changes in your life with greater ease.

To realize that the "Higher Power" is within you is very powerful, because it enables you to take responsibility for your own life. You can no longer see yourself as a "victim" who has no choice in your circumstances, because you have the answers within you to deal with any situation.

If you are in a situation that is uncomfortable or stressful, ask yourself, "Why am I allowing this to continue?" Perhaps you have made the *choice* to accept the consequences because of a benefit you hope to receive. If that is the case and you realize why you have made that choice, your inner spirit will see the whole situation from a different perspective. Then, you will be able to harvest the rewards of what you thought was a bad situation.

Or, you may realize that you don't have to endure the pain because of outside influences and you make a *choice* to remove yourself from the situation. Perhaps that situation was the catalyst to move you in a direction that is more constructive and beneficial to you.

In either case, you have made the choice — not someone else!

When you take responsibility for your life through the realization that you live with the guidance of your Spiritual Higher Self, you also realize that you have the *choice* to make your life what you want it to be.

Drop all the *shoulds, could haves, would haves* that are created by society and the environment you live in and take a real in-depth look at what your honest desires are. Ask yourself what makes you happy and content. By developing your awareness of your "Higher Self," "The God within you," you will find that all the answers you seek, to make your life the best it can be, lie within you. No one else can give you the answers that work for you and, likewise, you do not have the answers for someone else's life.

The loving purity of your Spiritual Higher Power will guide you in the right direction if you listen to it.

The happiness you achieve is accompanied by love and acceptance for all humanity because you are bonded by the common thread of life. To live without judgment of others is truly a spiritual freedom that enables you to rise above the guilt and false images that sometimes get in the way of seeing each other for who we really are.

When you can give up your judgment of others, you will find it easier to give up judgment of yourself. *That is the greatest freedom!*

You are entitled to whatever you desire for your happiness because we are all created with the same elements that connect a human being to the Universal Power, to "God," or whatever name you want to use. Joy and fulfillment are your divine birthright and the essence of your life. To be sure, life is full of problems to solve, but how you deal with them is what will make your life either happy or stressful.

Are you negative, believing that bad things happen to destroy your quality of life? Cast out all thoughts of negativity, they have never been known to solve a problem. Look to your Higher Self for the wisdom to guide you out of the dark and turn a bad situation into a positive resolution.

This is how you grow in wisdom and character. This is what makes your life rich and colorful. Problem solving is a challenge, a game that keeps you alert and informed. You are probably saying, "I would love to have a life without problems to solve." But, then you would have no need to grow, no feelings of accomplishment, no satisfaction in turning a negative into a positive, no participation in opening doors to a new and wonderful experience of Life. How boring your life, and you, would become.

Find Peace Within Yourself

Negativity is a destroyer of peace, happiness and love.

What will it matter how the world sees you if you don't feel good about yourself inside? A truly beautiful person, you, will be apparent to everyone when you develop a *positive or optimistic attitude* about yourself and the world around you. *Negativity* is a destroyer of peace, happiness and love.

Listed below are some tips to start you on your way towards realizing the zest and excitement of the life you are entitled to live.

1. Each day, take time to let go of limiting thought concepts. Don't be static, dull and inflexible.

Remember the children's story of the "Little Engine" who had to pull a long train of cars up a steep mountain. As long as he believed it was an impossible task — it was! When he decided to see it as a possibility, saying, "I think I can" — it started to become a reality. And as he continued in the confidence of "I think I can," each inch of progress led him to believe — "I know I can!" Yes, there were times when the train slid backwards, but he persevered and never doubted his ability to conquer and he reached his goal.

Be open to ongoing levels of truth. Each setback is only another opportunity for you to investigate and grow. When you can realize what is happening and accept the truth of what part you played in making it happen, you will be aware of the steps you must take to get on with your life. Only you can give yourself permission to move forward with what would make you happy and fulfilled.

2. For one half-hour each day, *study* the different methods (meditation, affirmations, self-help practices, religious values, introspection, etc.) that will bring about your self-awareness. When you understand their processes, practice them.

When I start my day with 15 minutes to ½ hr. of meditation and affirmations, I really see a difference in how I manage the obstacles I encounter throughout the day. I also apply these techniques before a very important audition or meeting. What a difference I experience in my body and mind. I approach the situation with a prepared, confident strength that would not have been there if I had not "centered" myself. This is actually getting in touch with my "Higher Self" and having faith that my best efforts will be present. If the outcome is not in my favor, I know that I presented my best and my performance was not at fault.

3. How many times have you or someone else said, " I don't know what I want in life, or what will make me happy." I have faced that dilemma many times, but realized that it would take some time and effort on my part to focus on where my path to happiness and fulfillment was meant to lead me.

For a start, make a list of your desires. Let your imagination go wild. You will think most of them are impossible to accomplish, but that is your limited, negative concept at work. Perhaps those dreams may not be attainable within a short period of time because of your present circumstances. *But,* they just might help you focus on a goal to work towards — step by step — a little bit each day. The secret to reaching a long distance goal is to set mini-goals that lead you on the path to the pot-of-gold at the end of the rainbow.

Make your goal something you really value and want. This will give you the motivation to continue when the going gets rough. For instance, your long-range goal is to own a house by the sea that costs $150,000. You or your husband make only $500 a week (after taxes) and you have no assets. Sounds impossible, doesn't it? Well, it isn't. The down-payment might be 10% or $15,000, maybe less if you can negotiate a lower price.

Write down everything you spend money on in one week that is not necessary for your survival, such as cigarettes, alcohol, entertainment, etc. Amazing how fast it adds up — probably $75 to $100. Now decide to bank or invest that money each week instead.

Set a mini-goal of $1,000 to be saved in ten weeks. (That's $100 a week that you would have spent on trivial amusements.) Now you are one step closer to getting your something of value to you. Continue for the next ten weeks, setting a goal of $2,000. Perhaps, you will find a little extra somewhere to bank, increasing your total. By the end of the year (52 weeks), you will have at least $5,200 plus interest and whatever additional monies you were able to put aside.

By working towards a short-term goal, you don't feel overwhelmed. You will gain encouragement as your balance grows and your motivation will become stronger. If that house really means something to you, you will probably find other ways to put money aside for your growing balance. Your accomplishment feeds your enthusiasm.

I have also experienced amazing results when I meditate and make affirmations for something I feel a strong desire to achieve. My Higher Power has opened doors I never would have thought possible and has revealed solutions for overcoming obstacles. When you have faith in your strengths, you can reach goals beyond your dreams.

4. Understand Life as Beauty, Truth, Wholeness, and Fulfillment. That is the way Life is meant to be for everyone. But it is not handed to you on a silver platter. The Game of Life is to encounter problems or obstacles and find a way to solve them. Life is a riddle and the feelings of power, self-esteem, excitement and satisfaction are the rewards for taking charge of your circumstance and turning it into a positive action towards your goal. Millions are made on games that are conceived and sold in the marketplace for your enjoyment — why not see your Life as a game that awaits you every morning that you awaken?!

5. Perceive Life as an eternal flow of energy — a constant movement through your body and mind and all around you — changing from moment to moment like the images on a movie screen. Life is always changing, be open and receptive to it. Put aside the racing thoughts of control and enjoy each moment, truly seeing and experiencing what is happening and realizing that there is a Higher Power flowing through your Life. As you relax into the rhythm of this flow of energy, you feel tension and frustration melting away. This is when the answers that are best for your happiness will become clear to you.

6. Communication with others is important so you can realize your connection to humanity. You are a sociable creature and need the balance of being with others, sharing the energy flow. You'll laugh, you'll cry, and you may even disagree with them. But remember, each person is entitled to their own perceptions and opinions so just listen and share. Your opinions and perceptions are not necessarily right for them. Through communication, you can discover parts of yourself that you may have forgotten or thought were not possible. This can be an enlightening experience and, in most cases, very satisfying. Sharing with others heightens the experience and gives you a sense of well-being and belonging.

Do not try to control or manipulate others to bring about your happiness. True happiness comes when you accept that you are subject to human frailties and you can love who you are unconditionally anyway. You are another human being trying to solve your everyday challenges in order

True happiness comes when you accept that you are subject to human frailties and you can love who you are anyway.

**Make
a list
of
your
good
traits.
Underline
your
best
ones.
This
will
remind
you
of how
wonderful
you
really
are.**

to capture the best experiences of your life. You will see others in a different perspective and feel love for them also. They, too, have challenges to overcome and they, too, seek the joys of their life. By realizing that you have the Spiritual Higher Power within you, just as everyone else has, you will see that *no one is better than you or less than you.* When you can honestly understand that, you will know that *self-esteem* is only a matter of being non-judgmental and accepting of others and, most of all, *of yourself.*

7. Make a list of your good traits. Underline what you feel are your best ones. This will remind you of how wonderful you really are. Put the list next to your bathroom mirror so you will start each day with a positive look at yourself. Remember, all human beings have the same qualities in them, but may have lost touch with these qualities because of circumstances they could not cope with. Have compassion.

8. It also gives you a great sense of satisfaction and belonging to be able to help others unconditionally, with a pure sense of giving and without any expectation of getting something in return. Volunteer to cook or bring food to the homeless. Form a group that brings music and entertainment to senior citizens, orphan homes, hospital wards, etc. If you have a hobby, perhaps you can teach it to a young person or anyone who would enjoy the activity. Create a program of your talents — cooking, sewing, decorating, etc. — and bring it to groups that are less fortunate than you. There are so many ways to reach out to others. It's amazing how giving of yourself gives you a sense of purpose and self-worth.

9. Read poetry — the romantic classics, Shakespeare, Haiku (a type of poetry that has purity and musical quality in its form). Read novels — romantic, science-fiction, mystery, foreign intrigue or any others that suit your interest. Reading stirs and enhances your imagination. It also offers an escape from feeling in a rut with everyday routines.

10. Now that your imagination has been stimulated — *write*! Try writing poetry, a novel, a daily diary, a letter to someone you have been out of touch with, or just write your thoughts about a situation that is predominant in your life. Thoughts are very fleeting, so keep a pad and pen nearby to record any that you want to preserve.

Seeing your thoughts on paper can help you determine what is important to you and can give you insight into who you really are. It can also help you solve problems. Creating something of your own can give you a great sense of satisfaction. And who knows, you might find a new avenue for fulfillment.

11. Try your hand at *art*. Drawing, painting, needlework, sewing. All are creative forms you do with your hands. It doesn't have to be museum quality or subject to anyone's judgment. The joy and satisfaction you can experience when you create with

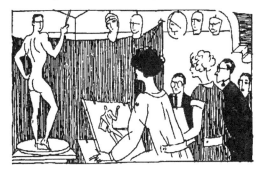

your hands will give you a sense of self-worth. There is also a very spiritual value to creating with your hands. It brings you to a place of tranquility, like a meditation with your spirit.

Gardening is also a form of art that puts you in touch with your spirituality. When you see the growth and blossoming of your efforts, you realize that, although you did the physical planting, there is a Higher Power which has joined forces with you to bring your efforts to life.

12. Music is a wonderful motivator. Different types of music can create an atmosphere that relaxes you, energizes you, or makes you happy or sad, and can definitely add to your spirituality. Music is very much connected to the rhythms and sounds of your life. You hear it differently from anyone else because it brings images and memories to your mind that only you have experienced or dreamed about. Listen to different types of music and use them to enhance your life.

When I hear Gregorian chants, religious music, sounds of nature, *The Grand Canyon Suite, Chariots of Fire* or other inspirational music, I feel the definitive presence of a Higher Power. I choose upbeat, rhythmic music to exercise with. When I need to relax, new-age instrumentals or classical music are my medicine. Music with "blue notes" will make me feel melancholy and bring me to tears.

13. Go a step further and learn to play an instrument. If you already play one, take up another. The motive behind this is to open your horizons and give you a new path to explore that will make you feel good about yourself. Create or join a group of fellow musicians, just for fun or with a goal in mind. This will also feed your need for social contact.

It is said that "Music hath powers to soothe the savage beast." Yes, music has great powers. Use it to your advantage.

14. Try *dancing*! This goes along with music. You have seen, or might have participated in the dancing that takes place in religious ceremonies. The movement of the body to the rhythm of the music can be the very spiritual experience of being one with the Higher Power. There is something very special about giving up all control and allowing the basic rhythms of life to take over.

On the other hand, dancing with a partner in a ballroom, club or in your own living room, can be very rewarding, too. It brings you closer to the feeling of being in harmony with another spirit.

Dancing is beneficial for toning the muscles of the body and is a very pleasant way to lose weight. Think of all the fun you can have just being in the atmosphere of people having fun and feeling good about themselves.

Embracing Change

Spirituality plays a major role in the evolution of your life. Realizing that there is a greater power than your conscious mind governing your life is the first step in accepting that change is inevitable throughout your life. All of creation is in a constant state of change.

For example, a tree begins life as a seed; struggles to become a sapling; blossoms with new life each spring; flourishes in the summer; loses its foliage each autumn; sleeps throughout the winter; then blossoms the following spring with fuller and richer vigor. Do you see the parallel to human life? There is a beginning, middle, and end to everything — and then another beginning — no matter how awesome or trivial. And, just as you experience the beauty of each stage of that tree's growth, the beauty of each stage of your growth is equally fascinating — if you allow yourself to appreciate the present.

Surviving The "Empty Nest"

Surviving the "empty nest"was very difficult for me because I tried to hold on to the happiness I had with the companionship of my two children while they were "under my wing." Also, while they were with me, it fulfilled my need to be needed. The more I tried to hold on, though, the more pain I experienced at the thought of losing them to someone else. And I must acknowledge the added pressure it must have put on them in their passage from childhood to adulthood. My fear of what might happen in the future kept me from fully enjoying what I had in the present.

When I realized my resistance to Change was doing more harm than good, I turned to my Inner Spirit for guidance. "Let go; don't stifle growth; accept change; new experiences lie ahead." The messages were coming loud and clear.

My faith in the positive action of life took over and I was able to relax into the flow of my next life chapter. To my amazement, I found a whole new, wonderful experience unfolding. My children spread their wings and got on with their lives, but they never "left" me. Instead, they have brought others into their lives who have multiplied my family, bringing even more love and joy than before. My life opened up to new avenues of fulfillment and I find it wildly exciting to have so much freedom to explore my desires while still enjoying the benefits of the love and happiness of my extended family. My newest chapter to explore is the realm of being a grandmother. My faith in the Spiritual Truths has never failed me.

Be still enough to listen to the guidance of your Intuition (your Higher Self), instead of holding on to "what is, " and each new experience will become richer and more meaning-ful. Have you ever been full of anxiety because you feared los-ing what you have, only to find that, when you let go, a new and more wonderful experience occurred? Many times it was much better than what you were holding onto. And, in many cases, you never lost what you had anyway, you only added more depth to your experience with the new addition.

Relationships — A New Life

Embracing changes in your relationships can bring new life to them. Love grows in many ways, bringing changes that you may not understand at the moment.

Any change in what you've become accustomed to can cause feelings of uneasiness and stress. Even the known neg-ative feelings can seem more comfortable than the risk of the unknown. Allow your Higher Power to guide you through the negative times. Remember, your human experiences have colored the way a situation appears to be, so if you honor your inner spiritual voice, you will find that you are where you need to be. You are on a transitional journey from old patterns that no longer work for you and those around you to a higher plateau in your life that will bring even greater joys.

Love is one of the strongest aspects of the feeling of wholeness. It is actually a spiritual need to feel complete and integrated. If you are searching for that need to be fulfilled by a mate, your children, your friends, or even in an abstract way by the people you work with — you are creating a potential source of unhappiness.

Looking to others for approval, recognition, rewards and romantic love only creates dependency and a feeling of being incomplete. That dependency creates fear of not getting what you want, rejection, unworthiness, internal conflict and loss. The fear makes you weigh and manipulate your interaction with others in order to gain that powerful feeling of oneness and worthiness. It becomes a losing battle because you are not coming from a place of self-love. You are not being true to yourself because you create images that you think will generate the love. Those images or false impressions cannot be sustained and eventually the real you surfaces. This creates confusion in your relationships and can eventually destroy your sense of well-being when the other person sees the real you as being false.

> Looking to others for approval, recognition, rewards, and romantic love only creates dependency and a feeling of being incomplete.

When you look for a mate or others to fulfill your need for love, you choose from a basic misconception. You may expect them to override your feelings of inadequacy and unworthiness but, if this is the case, you are selecting a mate for the wrong reasons. You will see them as your salvation because of a distorted perception of happiness and when your expectations are not fulfilled, you become disappointed and disillusioned, and blame them for your lack of happiness. You, in turn, are probably causing them great pain and confusion.

Your self-love has probably been attacked and altered by the many experiences you had as you grew from childhood to today. Your identity has been confused by unconscious fears of not being sufficient. The only way to get back to that wonderful, whole, spiritually complete being is to become conscious of who you really are.

True love can only be based on honesty with yourself. It must be self-sufficient and self-fulfilling. Not dependent on anyone. It is *spiritual*. It comes from your inner source — your Higher Power — the Divine within You.

When you love yourself, no one can make you feel unworthy, insufficient, incomplete. You are a complete unit within yourself. No one can take it away from you. That is what God intended you to be. A complete, self-fulfilling individual. You are love — created by the Master of Creation to exist as a complete individual in the realm of Humanity. Adam and Eve were created as complete individuals to share life — not to supply a missing essential in each other.

Face the fears that suppress your freedom to be who you really are. Confront any feelings of inadequacy you may have. Search for what created those feelings and recognize their source. Did you believe what you thought someone else's opinion of you was or did you misinterpret what they implied? No one really knows you as well as you do. And no one can be the judge of your motivations.

Your search may need the help of a professional or you may be able to dispel your fearful disclaimers by working through them by yourself, with the aid of the many self-help books on the market, seminars, or by just exploring the spiritual philosophies of your choice.

In any case, it is possible to overcome the monsters that sap your energy, distort your perception, cause you to make choices you don't want, and make you feel miserable and trapped in deceit.

When you learn to see yourself as a loving, self-accepting individual, you will be able to *share* your wonderful self with others — including a loving mate. What a wonderful, exciting and fulfilling experience it is to have the companionship of another complete individual. There are no false pretenses, no games — just pure happiness in enjoying each other and watching the ever-changing growth of another human being.

❖ *I have always heard it said that "you cannot give love unless you love yourself," and "you cannot accept another's love unless you can believe that you are lovable." Be a true friend to yourself. Nurture and love the confused child within you until you know that you are a wonderful, complete being. Let your loving spirit bring forth the unconditional acceptance of the beauty within you. Only then, will you openly and freely give love to those around you and recognize the truth in the love that is offered to you. That is the state of true happiness!*

—Vernice Gabriel

Index

A

abdominal cramps, 139

activated charcoal tablets, 134

acidophilus, 136

adrenal gland, 180

age spots, 367

alcohol, 44, 138, 153, 159-160, 180, 196, 213, 220, 228

alfalfa, 30, 209

algar, 205

almonds, 125, 176, 211

aluminum, 87-88, 160, 208, 214

anise seed, 159

antacids, 160

anti-depressants, 214

antibiotics, 214

antioxidants, 184-187, 258

apples, 30, 33, 100-101, 115, 125, 212

apricots, 115, 127, 188

arteriosclerosis, 123

arthritis, 57-80

   arthitis exercises, 71-78

   arthritis fighting herbs, 61

artichokes, 101, 114

asparagus, 43, 114

asthma, 81-96

astragalus, 193

avocados, 63, 147, 175

B

backaches, 111

bananas, 115, 136, 147, 159, 175

barbiturates, 214

barley, 101, 113, 212, 249

beans, 63, 100, 114, 124, 147, 163, 175, 176, 206, 230, 240, 244

bee pollen, 44

beef, 43, 102, 147, 175, 187, 194, 222, 250

C

O

P

𝒯